BASES OF YOGA

BASES DE YOGA

Sri Aurobindo

BASES OF YOGA

LOTUS LIGHT PUBLICATIONS
Box 325, Twin Lakes, WI 53181
USA

Published and distributed in the United States by
Lotus Light Publications, Box 325, Twin Lakes, WI 53181
by arrangement with Sri Aurobindo Ashram Trust,
Publication Department, Pondicherry 605 002, India

First U.S. edition 1993

ISBN: 0-941524-77-9
Library of Congress Catalog Card Number: 93-79795

Printed at the Sri Aurobindo Ashram Press,
Pondicherry, India

PRINTED IN INDIA

Publishers' Note

These are extracts from letters written by Sri Aurobindo to his disciples in answer to their queries. They have been put together and arranged so as to be of some help to aspirants for the understanding and practice of the Yoga.

CONTENTS

I

CALM – PEACE – EQUALITY

It is not possible to make a foundation in Yoga if the mind is restless. The first thing needed is quiet in the mind. Also to merge the personal consciousness is not the first aim of the Yoga: the first aim is to open it to a higher spiritual consciousness and for this also a quiet mind is the first need.

*

The first thing to do in the sadhana is to get a settled peace and silence in the mind. Otherwise you may have experiences, but nothing will be permanent. It is in the silent mind that the true consciousness can be built.

A quiet mind does not mean that there will be no thoughts or mental movements at all, but that these will be on the surface and you will feel your true being within separate from them, observing but not carried away, able to watch and judge them and reject all that has to be rejected and to accept and keep to all that is true consciousness and true experience.

Passivity of the mind is good, but take care to be passive only to the Truth and to the touch of the Divine Shakti. If you are passive to the suggestions and influences of the lower nature, you will not be able to progress or else you will expose yourself to adverse forces which may take you far away from the true path of Yoga.

Aspire to the Mother for this settled quietness and calm of the mind and this constant sense of the inner being in you standing back from the external nature and turned to the Light and Truth.

The forces that stand in the way of sadhana are the forces of the lower mental, vital and physical nature. Behind them are adverse powers of the mental, vital and subtle physical worlds. These can be dealt with only after the mind and heart have become one-pointed and concentrated in the single aspiration to the Divine.

*

Silence is always good; but I do not mean by quietness of mind entire silence. I mean a mind free from disturbance and trouble, steady, light and glad so as to open to the Force that will change the nature. The important thing is to get rid of the habit of the invasion of troubling thoughts, wrong feelings, confusion of ideas, unhappy movements. These disturb the nature and cloud it and make it difficult for the Force to work; when the mind is quiet and at peace, the Force can work more easily. It should be possible to see things that have to be changed in you without being upset or depressed; the change is the more easily done.

*

The difference between a vacant mind and a calm mind is this: that when the mind is vacant, there is no thought, no conception, no mental action of any kind, except an essential perception of things without the formed idea; but in the calm mind, it is the substance of the mental being that is still, so still that nothing disturbs it. If thoughts or activities come, they do not rise at all out of the mind, but they come from outside and cross the mind as a flight of birds crosses the sky in a windless air. It passes, disturbs nothing, leaving no trace. Even if a thousand images or the most violent events pass across it, the calm stillness remains as if the very texture of the mind were a substance of eternal and indestructible peace. A mind that has achieved this calmness can begin to act, even intensely and powerfully, but it will keep its fundamental stillness – originating nothing from itself but receiving from Above and giving it a mental form without adding anything of its own, calmly, dispassionately, though with the joy of the Truth and the happy power and light of its passage.

*

It is not an undesirable thing for the mind to fall silent, to be free from thoughts and still – for it is oftenest when the mind falls silent that there is the full descent of a wide peace from above and in that wide tranquillity the realisation of the silent Self above the mind spread out in its vastness everywhere. Only, when there is the peace and the mental silence, the vital mind tries to rush in and occupy the place or else the mechanical mind tries to raise up for the same purpose its round of trivial habitual thoughts. What the sadhak has to do is to be careful to reject and hush these outsiders, so that during the meditation at least the peace and quietude of the mind and vital may be complete. This can be done best if you keep a strong and silent will. That will is the will of the Purusha behind the mind; when the mind is at peace, when it is silent one can become aware of the Purusha, silent also, separate from the action of the nature.

To be calm, steady, fixed in the spirit, *dhīra sthira*, this quietude of the mind, this separation of the inner Purusha from the outer Prakriti is very helpful, almost indispen-

sable. So long as the being is subject to the whirl of
thoughts or the turmoil of the vital movements, one cannot be thus calm and fixed in the spirit. To detach oneself,
to stand back from them, to feel them separate from
oneself is indispensable.

For the discovery of the true individuality and building
up of it in the nature, two things are necessary, first, to be
conscious of one's psychic being behind the heart and,
next, this separation of the Purusha from the Prakriti. For
the true individual is behind veiled by the activities of the
outer nature.

*

A great wave (or sea) of calm and the constant consciousness of a vast and luminous Reality – this is precisely the
character of the fundamental realisation of the Supreme
Truth in its first touch on the mind and the soul. One
could not ask for a better beginning or foundation – it is
like a rock on which the rest can be built. It means
certainly not only a Presence, but *the* Presence – and it
would be a great mistake to weaken the experience by any
non-acceptance or doubt of its character.

It is not necessary to define it and one ought not even to
try to turn it into an image; for this Presence is in its
nature infinite. Whatever it has to manifest of itself or out
of itself, it will do inevitably by its own power, if there is a
sustained acceptance.

It is quite true that it is a grace sent and the only return
needed for such a grace is acceptance, gratitude and to
allow the Power that has touched the consciousness to
develop what has to be developed in the being – by keeping oneself open to it. The total transformation of the

nature cannot be done in a moment; it must take long and proceed through stages; what is now experienced is only an initiation, a foundation for the new consciousness in which that transformation will become possible. The automatic spontaneity of the experience ought by itself to show that it is nothing constructed by the mind, will or emotions; it comes from a Truth that is beyond them.

*

To reject doubts means control of one's thoughts – very certainly so. But the control of one's thoughts is as necessary as the control of one's vital desires and passions or the control of the movements of one's body – for the Yoga, and not for the Yoga only. One cannot be a fully developed mental being even, if one has not a control of the thoughts, is not their observer, judge, master, – the mental Purusha, *manomaya puruṣa, sākṣī, anumantā, īśvara.* It is no more proper for the mental being to be the tennis-ball of unruly and uncontrollable thoughts than to be a rudderless ship in the storm of the desires and passions or a slave of either the inertia or the impulses of the body. I know it is more difficult because man being primarily a creature of mental Prakriti identifies himself with the movements of his mind and cannot at once dissociate himself and stand free from the swirl and eddies of the mind whirlpool. It is comparatively easy for him to put a control on his body, at least on a certain part of its movements; it is less easy but still very possible after a struggle to put a mental control on his vital impulsions and desires; but to sit like the Tantric Yogi on the river, above the whirlpool of his thoughts, is less facile. Nevertheless, it can be done; all developed mental men, those who get beyond the average, have in one way or other or at least at certain times and for certain purposes to separate the two parts of the mind, the active part which is a factory of thoughts and the quiet masterful part which is at once a Witness and a Will, observing them, judging, rejecting, eliminating, accepting, ordering corrections and changes, the Master in the House of Mind, capable of self-empire, *sāmrājya*.

The Yogi goes still farther; he is not only a master there, but even while in mind in a way, he gets out of it as it were, and stands above or quite back from it and free. For him the image of the factory of thoughts is no longer quite valid; for he sees that thoughts come from outside, from the universal Mind or universal Nature, sometimes formed and distinct, sometimes unformed and then they are given shape somewhere in us. The principal business of our mind is either a response of acceptance or a refusal to these thought-waves (as also vital waves, subtle physical energy waves) or this giving personal-mental form to thought-stuff (or vital movements) from the environing Nature-Force.

The possibilities of the mental being are not limited, it can be the free Witness and Master in its own house. A progressive freedom and mastery over one's mind is perfectly within the possibilities of anyone who has faith and will to undertake it.

*

The first step is a quiet mind – silence is a further step, but quietude must be there; and by a quiet mind I mean a mental consciousness within, which sees thoughts arrive to it and move about but does not itself feel that it is thinking or identifying itself with the thoughts or call them its own. Thoughts, mental movements may pass through it as way-farers appear and pass from elsewhere through a silent country – the quiet mind observes them or does not care to observe them, but, in either case, does not become active or lose its quietude. Silence is more than quietude; it can be gained by banishing thought altogether from the inner mind, keeping it voiceless or quite outside; but more easily it is established by a descent from above – one feels it coming down, entering and occupying or surrounding the personal consciousness which then tends to merge itself in the vast impersonal silence.

*

The words "peace, calm, quiet, silence" have each their own shade of meaning, but it is not easy to define them.

Peace – *śānti*.
Calm – *sthiratā*.
Quiet – *acañcalatā*.
Silence – *niścala nīravatā*.

Quiet is a condition in which there is no restlessness or disturbance.

Calm is a still unmoved condition which no disturbance can affect – it is a less negative condition than quiet.

Peace is a still more positive condition; it carries with it a sense of settled and harmonious rest and deliverance.

Silence is a state in which either there is no movement of the mind or vital or else a great stillness which no surface movement can pierce or alter.

*

Keep the quietude and do not mind if it is for a time an empty quietude; the consciousness is often like a vessel which has to be emptied of its mixed or undesirable contents; it has to be kept vacant for a while till it can be filled with things new and true, right and pure. The one thing to be avoided is the refilling of the cup with the old turbid contents. Meanwhile wait, open yourself upwards, call very quietly and steadily, not with a too restless eagerness, for the peace to come into the silence and, once the peace is there, for the joy and the presence.

*

Calm, even if it seems at first only a negative thing, is so difficult to attain, that to have it at all must be regarded as a great step in advance.

In reality, calm is not a negative thing, it is the very nature of the Sat-Purusha and the positive foundation of the divine consciousness. Whatever else is aspired for and gained, this must be kept. Even Knowledge, Power, Ananda, if they come and do not find this foundation, are unable to remain and have to withdraw until the divine purity and peace of the Sat-Purusha are permanently there.

Aspire for the rest of the divine consciousness, but with a calm and deep aspiration. It can be ardent as well as calm, but not impatient, restless or full of rajasic eagerness.

Only in the quiet mind and being can the supramental Truth build its true creation.

*

Experience in the sadhana is bound to begin with the mental plane, – all that is necessary is that the experience should be sound and genuine. The pressure of understanding and will in the mind and the Godward emotional urge in the heart are the two first agents of Yoga, and peace, purity and calm (with a lulling of the lower unrest) are precisely the first basis that has to be laid; to get that is much more important in the beginning than to get a glimpse of the supraphysical worlds or to have visions, voices and powers. Purification and calm are the first needs in the Yoga. One may have a great wealth of experiences of that kind (worlds, visions, voices, etc.) without them, but these experiences occurring in an unpurified and troubled consciousness are usually full of disorder and mixture.

At first the peace and calm are not continuous, they come and go, and it usually takes a long time to get them settled in the nature. It is better therefore to avoid impatience and to go on steadily with what is being done. If you wish to have something beyond the peace and calm, let it be the full opening of the inner being and the consciousness of the Divine Power working in you. Aspire for that sincerely and with a great intensity but without impatience and it will come.

*

At last you have the true foundation of the sadhana. This calm, peace and surrender are the right atmosphere for all the rest to come, knowledge, strength, Ananda. Let it become complete.

It does not remain when engaged in work because it is still confined to the mind proper which has only just received the gift of silence. When the new consciousness is fully formed and has taken entire possession of the vital nature and the physical being (the vital as yet is only touched or dominated by the silence, not possessed by it), then this defect will disappear.

The quiet consciousness of peace you now have in the mind must become not only calm but wide. You must feel it everywhere, yourself in it and all in it. This also will help to bring the calm as a basis into the action.

The wider your consciousness becomes, the more you will be able to receive from above. The Shakti will be able to descend and bring strength and light as well as peace into the system. What you feel as narrow and limited in you is the physical mind; it can only widen if this wider consciousness and the light come down and possess the nature.

The physical inertia from which you suffer is likely to lessen and disappear only when strength from above descends into the system.

Remain quiet, open yourself and call the divine Shakti to confirm the calm and peace, to widen the consciousness and to bring into it as much light and power as it can at present receive and assimilate.

Take care not to be over-eager, as this may disturb again such quiet and balance as has been already established in the vital nature.

Have confidence in the final result and give time for the Power to do its work.

*

Aspire, concentrate in the right spirit and, whatever the difficulties, you are sure to attain the aim you have put before you.

It is in the peace behind and that "something truer" in you that you must learn to live and feel it to be yourself. You must regard the rest as not your real self, but only a flux of changing or recurring movements on the surface which are sure to go as the true self emerges.

Peace is the true remedy; distraction by hard work is only a temporary relief – although a certain amount of work is necessary for the proper balance of the different parts of the being. To feel the peace above and about your head is a first step; you have to get connected with it and it must descend into you and fill your mind and life and body and surround you so that you live in it – for this peace is the one sign of the Divine's presence with you, and once you have it all the rest will begin to come.

Truth in speech and truth in thought are very important. The more you can feel falsehood as being not part of yourself, as coming on you from outside, the easier it will be to reject and refuse it.

Persevere and what is still crooked will be made straight and you will know and feel constantly the truth of the Divine's presence and your faith will be justified by direct experience.

*

First aspire and pray to the Mother for quiet in the mind, purity, calm and peace, an awakened consciousness, intensity of devotion, strength and spiritual capacity to face all inner and outer difficulties and go through to the end of the Yoga. If the consciousness awakens and there is devotion and intensity of aspiration, it will be possible for the mind, provided it learns quietude and peace, to grow in knowledge.

*

This is due to an acute consciousness and sensitiveness of the physical being, especially the vital-physical.

It is good for the physical to be more and more conscious, but it should not be over-powered by these ordinary human reactions of which it becomes aware or badly affected or upset by them. A strong equality and mastery and detachment must come, in the nerves and body as in the mind, which will enable the physical to know and contact these things without feeling any disturbance; it should know and be conscious and reject and throw away the pressure of the movements in the atmosphere, not merely feel them and suffer.

*

To recognise one's weaknesses and false movements and draw back from them is the way towards liberation.

Not to judge anyone but oneself until one can see things from a calm mind and a calm vital is an excellent rule. Also, do not allow your mind to form hasty impressions on the strength of some outward appearance, nor your vital to act upon them.

There is a place in the inner being where one can always remain calm and from there look with poise and judgment on the perturbations of the surface consciousness and act upon it to change it. If you can learn to live in that calm of the inner being, you will have found your stable basis.

*

Do not allow yourself to be shaken or troubled by these things. The one thing to do always is to remain firm in your aspiration to the Divine and to face with equanimity and detachment all difficulties and all oppositions. For those who wish to lead the spiritual life, the Divine must always come first, everything else must be secondary.

Keep yourself detached and look at these things from the calm inner vision of one who is inwardly dedicated to the Divine.

*

At present your experiences are on the mental plane, but that is the right movement. Many sadhaks are unable to advance because they open the vital plane before the mental and psychic are ready. After some beginning of true spiritual experiences on the mental plane there is a premature descent into the vital and great confusion and disturbance. This has to be guarded against. It is still worse if the vital desire-soul opens to experience before the mind has been touched by the things of the spirit.

Aspire always for the mind and psychic being to be filled with the true consciousness and experience and made ready. You must aspire especially for quietness, peace, a calm faith, an increasing steady wideness, for more and more knowledge, for a deep and intense but quiet devotion.

Do not be troubled by your surroundings and their opposition. These conditions are often imposed at first as a kind of ordeal. If you can remain tranquil and undisturbed and continue your sadhana without allowing yourself to be inwardly troubled under these circumstances, it will help to give you a much needed strength; for the path of Yoga is always beset with inner and outer difficulties and the sadhak must develop a quiet, firm and solid strength to meet them.

The inner spiritual progress does not depend on outer conditions so much as on the way we react to them from within – that has always been the ultimate verdict of spiritual experience. It is why we insist on taking the right attitude and persisting in it, on an inner state not dependent on outer circumstances, a state of equality and calm, if it cannot be at once of inner happiness, on going more and more within and looking from within outwards instead of living in the surface mind which is always at the mercy of the shocks and blows of life. It is only from that inner state that one can be stronger than life and its disturbing forces and hope to conquer.

To remain quiet within, firm in the will to go through, refusing to be disturbed or discouraged by difficulties or fluctuations, that is one of the first things to be learned in the Path. To do otherwise is to encourage the instability of consciousness, the difficulty of keeping experience of which you complain. It is only if you keep quiet and steady within that the lines of experience can go on with some steadiness – though they are never without periods of interruption and fluctuation; but these, if properly treated, can then become periods of assimilation and exhaustion of difficulty rather than denials of sadhana.

A spiritual atmosphere is more important than outer conditions; if one can get that and also create one's own spiritual air to breathe in and live in it, that is the true condition of progress.

*

To be able to receive the Divine Power and let it act through you in the things of the outward life, there are three necessary conditions:

(*i*) Quietude, equality – not to be disturbed by anything that happens, to keep the mind still and firm, seeing the play of forces, but itself tranquil.

(*ii*) Absolute faith – faith that what is for the best will happen, but also that if one can make oneself a true instrument, the fruit will be that which one's will guided by the Divine Light sees as the thing to be done – *kartavyam karma.*

(*iii*) Receptivity – the power to receive the Divine Force and to feel its presence and the presence of the Mother in it and allow it to work, guiding one's sight and will and action. If this power and presence can be felt and this plasticity made the habit of the consciousness in action, – but plasticity to the Divine Force alone without bringing in any foreign element, – the eventual result is sure.

*

Equality is a very important part of this Yoga; it is necessary to keep equality under pain and suffering – and that means to endure firmly and calmly, not to be restless or troubled or depressed or despondent, to go on with a steady faith in the Divine Will. But equality does not include inert acceptance. If, for instance, there is temporary failure of some endeavour in the sadhana, one has to keep equality, not to be troubled or despondent, but one has not to accept the failure as an indication of the Divine Will and give up the endeavour. You ought rather to find out the reason and meaning of the failure and go forward in faith towards victory. So with illness – you have not to be troubled, shaken or restless, but you have not to accept illness as the Divine Will, but rather look upon it as an imperfection of the body to be got rid of as you try to get rid of vital imperfections or mental errors.

*

There can be no firm foundation in sadhana without equality, *samatā*. Whatever the unpleasantness of circumstances, however disagreeable the conduct of others, you must learn to receive them with a perfect calm and without any disturbing reaction. These things are the test of equality. It is easy to be calm and equal when things go well and people and circumstances are pleasant; it is when they are the opposite that the completeness of the calm, peace, equality can be tested, reinforced, made perfect.

*

What happened to you shows what are the conditions of that state in which the Divine Power takes the place of the ego and directs the action, making the mind, life and body an instrument. A receptive silence of the mind, an effacement of the mental ego and the reduction of the mental being to the position of a witness, a close contact with the Divine Power and an openness of the being to that one Influence and no other are the conditions for becoming an instrument of the Divine, moved by that and that only.

The silence of the mind does not of itself bring in the supramental consciousness; there are many states or planes or levels of consciousness between the human mind and the Supermind. The silence opens the mind and the rest of the being to greater things, sometimes to the cosmic consciousness, sometimes to the experience of the silent Self,

sometimes to the presence or power of the Divine, sometimes to a higher consciousness than that of the human
mind; the mind's silence is the most favourable condition
for any of these things to happen. In this Yoga it is the
most favourable condition (not the only one) for the
Divine Power to descend first upon and then into the
individual consciousness and there do its work to transform that consciousness, giving it the necessary experiences, altering all its outlook and movements, leading it
from stage to stage till it is ready for the last (supramental)
change.

*

The experience of this "solid block" feeling indicates
the descent of a solid strength and peace into the external
being – but into the vital-physical most. It is this always
that is the foundation, the sure basis into which all else
(Ananda, light, knowledge, Bhakti) can descend in the
future and stand on it or play safely. The numbness was
there in the other experience because the movement
was inward; but here the Yogashakti is coming *outward*
into the fully aware external nature, – as a first step
towards the establishment of the Yoga and its experience
there. So the numbness which was a sign of the consciousness tending to draw back from the external parts is not
there.

*

Remember first that an inner quietude, caused by the
purification of the restless mind and vital, is the first
condition of a secure sadhana. Remember next, that to

feel the Mother's presence while in external action is already a great step and one that cannot be attained without a considerable inner progress. Probably, what you feel you need so much but cannot define is a constant and vivid sense of the Mother's force working in you, descending from above and taking possession of the different planes of your being. That is often a prior condition for the twofold movement of ascent and descent; it will surely come in time. These things can take a long time to begin visibly, especially when the mind is accustomed to be very active and has not the habit of mental silence. When that veiling activity is there, much work has to be carried on behind the mobile screen of the mind and the sadhak thinks nothing is happening when really much preparation is being done. If you want a more swift and visible progress, it can only be by bringing your psychic to the front through a constant self-offering. Aspire intensely, but without impatience.

*

A strong mind and body and life-force are needed in the sadhana. Especially steps should be taken to throw out tamas and bring strength and force into the frame of the nature.

The way of Yoga must be a living thing, not a mental principle or a set method to be stuck to against all necessary variations.

*

Not to be disturbed, to remain quiet and confident is the right attitude, but it is necessary also to receive the help of the Mother and not to stand back for any reason from her solicitude. One ought not to indulge ideas of incapacity, inability to respond, dwelling too much on defects and failures and allowing the mind to be in pain and shame on their account; for these ideas and feelings become in the end weakening things. If there are difficulties, stumblings or failures, one has to look at them quietly and call in tranquilly and persistently the Divine help for their removal, but not to allow oneself to be upset or pained or discouraged. Yoga is not an easy path and the total change of the nature cannot be done in a day.

*

The depression and vital struggle must have been due to some defect of over-eagerness and straining for a result in your former effort – so that when a fall in the consciousness came, it was a distressed, disappointed and confused vital that came to the surface giving full entry to the suggestions of doubt, despair and inertia from the adverse side of Nature. You have to move towards a firm basis of calm and equality in the vital and physical no less than in the mental consciousness; let there be the full downflow of Power and Ananda, but into a firm Adhar capable of containing it – it is complete equality that gives that capacity and firmness.

*

Wideness and calmness are the foundation of the Yogic consciousness and the best condition for inner growth and experience. If a wide calm can be established in the physical consciousness, occupying and filling the very body and all its cells, that can become the basis for its transformation; in fact, without this wideness and calmness the transformation is hardly possible.

*

It is the aim of the sadhana that the consciousness should rise out of the body and take its station above, – spreading in the wideness everywhere, not limited to the body. Thus liberated one opens to all that is above this station, above the ordinary mind, receives there all that descends from the heights, observes from there all that is below. Thus it is possible to witness in all freedom and to control all that is below and to be a recipient or a channel for all that comes down and presses into the body, which it will prepare to be an instrument of a higher manifestation, remoulded into a higher consciousness and nature.

What is happening in you is that the consciousness is trying to fix itself in this liberation. When one is there in that higher station, one finds the freedom of the Self and the vast silence and immutable calm – but this calm has to be brought down also into the body, into all the lower planes and fix itself there as something standing behind and containing all the movements.

*

If your consciousness rises above the head, that means that it goes beyond the ordinary mind to the centre above which receives the higher consciousness or else towards the ascending levels of the higher consciousness itself. The first result is the silence and peace of the Self which is the basis of the higher consciousness; this may afterwards descend into the lower levels, into the very body. Light also can descend and Force. The navel and the centres below it are those of the vital and the physical; something of the higher force may have descended there.

II

FAITH – ASPIRATION – SURRENDER

This Yoga demands a total dedication of the life to the aspiration for the discovery and embodiment of the Divine truth and to nothing else whatever. To divide your life between the Divine and some outward aim and activity that has nothing to do with the search for the Truth is inadmissible. The least thing of that kind would make success in the Yoga impossible.

You must go inside yourself and enter into a complete dedication to the spiritual life. All clinging to mental preferences must fall away from you, all insistence on vital aims and interests and attachments must be put away, all egoistic clinging to family, friends, country must disappear if you want to succeed in Yoga. Whatever has to come as outgoing energy or action, must proceed from the Truth once discovered and not from the lower mental or vital motives, from the Divine Will and not from personal choice or the preferences of the ego.

*

Mental theories are of no fundamental importance, for the mind forms or accepts the theories that support the turn of the being. What is important is that turn and the call within you.

The knowledge that there is a Supreme Existence, Consciousness and Bliss which is not merely a negative Nirvana or a static and featureless Absolute, but dynamic, the perception that this Divine Consciousness can be realised not only beyond but here, and the consequent acceptance of a divine life as the aim of Yoga, do not belong to the mind. It is not a question of mental theory – even though mentally this outlook can be as well supported as any other, if not better, – but of experience and, before the experience comes, of the soul's faith bringing with it the mind's and the life's adhesion. One who is in contact with the higher Light and has the experience can follow this way, however difficult it may be for the lower members to follow; one who is touched by it, without having the experience, but having the call, the conviction, the compulsion of the soul's adherence, can also follow it.

*

The ways of the Divine are not like those of the human mind or according to our patterns and it is impossible to judge them or to lay down for Him what He shall or shall not do, for the Divine knows better than we can know. If we admit the Divine at all, both true reason and bhakti seem to me to be at one in demanding implicit faith and surrender.

*

Not to impose one's mind and vital will on the Divine but to receive the Divine's will and follow it, is the true attitude of sadhana. Not to say, "This is my right, want, claim, need, requirement, why do I not get it?" but to give oneself, to surrender and to receive with joy whatever the Divine gives, not grieving or revolting, is the better way. Then what you receive will be the right thing for you.

*

Faith, reliance upon God, surrender and self-giving to the Divine Power are necessary and indispensable. But reliance upon God must not be made an excuse for indolence, weakness and surrender to the impulses of the lower Nature: it must go along with untiring aspiration and a persistent rejection of all that comes in the way of the Divine Truth. The surrender to the Divine must not be turned into an excuse, a cloak or an occasion for surrender to one's own desires and lower movements or to one's ego or to some Force of the ignorance and darkness that puts on a false appearance of the Divine.

*

You have only to aspire, to keep yourself open to the Mother, to reject all that is contrary to her will and to let her work in you – doing also all your work for her and in the faith that it is through her force that you can do it. If you remain open in this way the knowledge and realisation will come to you in due course.

*

In this Yoga all depends on whether one can open to the Influence or not. If there is a sincerity in the aspiration and a patient will to arrive at the higher consciousness in spite of all obstacles, then the opening in one form or another is sure to come. But it may take a long or short time according to the prepared or unprepared condition of the mind, heart and body; so if one has not the necessary patience, the effort may be abandoned owing to the difficulty of the beginning. There is no method in this Yoga except to concentrate, preferably in the heart, and call the presence and power of the Mother to take up the being and by the workings of her force transform the consciousness; one can concentrate also in the head or between the eyebrows, but for many this is a too difficult opening. When the mind falls quiet and the concentration becomes strong and the aspiration intense, then there is a beginning of experience. The more the faith, the more rapid the result is likely to be. For the rest one must not depend on one's own efforts only, but succeed in establishing a contact with the Divine and a receptivity to the Mother's Power and Presence.

*

It does not matter what defects you may have in your nature. The one thing that matters is your keeping yourself open to the Force. Nobody can transform himself by his own unaided efforts; it is only the Divine Force that can transform him. If you keep yourself open, all the rest will be done for you.

*

Hardly anyone is strong enough to overcome by his own unaided aspiration and will the forces of the lower nature; even those who do it get only a certain kind of control, but not a complete mastery. Will and aspiration are needed to bring down the aid of the Divine Force and to keep the being on its side in its dealings with the lower powers. The Divine Force fulfilling the spiritual will and the heart's psychic aspiration can alone bring about the conquest.

*

To do anything by mental control is always difficult, when what is attempted runs contrary to the trend of human nature or of the personal nature. A strong will patiently and perseveringly turned towards its object can effect a change, but usually it takes a long time and the success at the beginning may be only partial and chequered by many failures.

To turn all actions automatically into worship cannot be done by thought control only; there must be a strong aspiration in the heart which will bring about some realisation or feeling of the presence of the One to whom worship is offered. The bhakta does not rely on his own effort alone, but on the grace and power of the Divine whom he adores.

*

There has always been too much reliance on the action of your own mind and will – that is why you cannot progress. If you could once get the habit of silent reliance on the power of the Mother, – not merely calling it in to support your own effort, – the obstacle would diminish and eventually disappear.

*

All sincere aspiration has its effect; if you are sincere you will grow into the divine life.

To be entirely sincere means to desire the divine Truth only, to surrender yourself more and more to the Divine Mother, to reject all personal demand and desire other than this one aspiration, to offer every action in life to the Divine and do it as the work given without bringing in the ego. This is the basis of the divine life.

One cannot become altogether this at once, but if one aspires at all times and calls in always the aid of the Divine Shakti with a true heart and straightforward will, one grows more and more into this consciousness.

*

A complete surrender is not possible in so short a time, – for a complete surrender means to cut the knot of the ego in each part of the being and offer it, free and whole, to the Divine. The mind, the vital, the physical consciousness (and even each part of these in all its movements) have one after the other to surrender separately, to give up their own way and to accept the way of the Divine. But what one can do is to make from the beginning a central resolve and self-dedication and to implement it in whatever way one finds open, at each step, taking advantage of each occasion that offers itself to make the self-giving complete. A surrender in one direction makes others easier, more inevitable; but it does not of itself cut or loosen the other knots, and especially those which are very intimately bound up with the present personality and its most cherished formations may often present great difficulties, even after the central will has been fixed and the first seals put on its resolve in practice.

*

You ask how you can repair the wrong you seem to have done. Admitting that it is as you say, it seems to me that the reparation lies precisely in this, in making yourself a vessel for the Divine Truth and the Divine Love. And the first steps towards that are a complete self-consecration and self-purification, a complete opening of oneself to the Divine, rejecting all in oneself that can stand in the way of the fulfilment. In the spiritual life there is no other reparation for any mistake, none that is wholly effective. At the beginning one should not ask for any other fruit or results than this internal growth and change, – for otherwise one lays oneself open to severe disappointments. Only when one is free, can one free others and in Yoga it is out of the inner victory that there comes the outer conquest.

*

It is not possible to get rid of the stress on personal effort at once – and not always desirable; for personal effort is better than tamasic inertia.

The personal effort has to be transformed progressively into a movement of the Divine Force. If you feel conscious of the Divine Force, then call it in more and more to govern your effort, to take it up, to transform it into something not yours, but the Mother's. There will be a sort of transfer, a taking up of the forces at work in the personal Adhar – a transfer not suddenly complete but progressive.

But the psychic poise is necessary: the discrimination must develop which sees accurately what is the Divine Force, what is the element of personal effort, and what is brought in as a mixture from the lower cosmic forces. And until the transfer is complete which always takes time, there must always be as a personal contribution, a constant consent to the true Force, a constant rejection of any lower mixture.

At present to give up personal effort is not what is

wanted, but to call in more and more the Divine Power and govern and guide by it the personal endeavour.

*

It is not advisable in the early stages of the sadhana to leave everything to the Divine or expect everything from it without the need of one's own endeavour. That is only possible when the psychic being is in front and influencing the whole action (and even then vigilance and a constant assent are necessary), or else later on in the ultimate stages of the Yoga when a direct or almost direct supramental force is taking up the consciousness; but this stage is very far away as yet. Under other conditions this attitude is likely to lead to stagnation and inertia.

It is only the more mechanical parts of the being that can truly say they are helpless: the physical (material) consciousness, especially, is inert in its nature and moved either by the mental and vital or by the higher forces. But one has always the power to put the mental will or vital push at the service of the Divine. One cannot be sure of the immediate result, for the obstruction of the lower Nature or the pressure of the adverse forces can often act successfully for a time, even for a long time, against the necessary change. One has then to persist, to put always the will on the side of the divine, rejecting what has to be rejected, opening oneself to the true Light and the true Force, calling it down quietly, steadfastly, without tiring, without depression or impatience, until one feels the Divine Force at work and the obstacles beginning to give way.

You say you are conscious of your ignorance and obscurity. If it is only a general consciousness, that is not enough.

But if you are conscious of it in the details, in its actual working, then that is sufficient to start with; you have to reject steadfastly the wrong workings of which you are conscious and make your mind and vital a quiet and clear field for the action of the Divine Force.

*

The mechanical movements are always more difficult to stop by the mental will, because they do not in the least depend upon reason or any mental justification but are founded upon association or else a mere mechanical memory and habit.

The practice of rejection prevails in the end; but with personal effort only, it may take a long time. If you can feel the Divine Power working in you, then it should become easier.

There should be nothing inert or tamasic in the self-giving to the guidance and it should not be made by any part of the vital into a plea for not rejecting the suggestions of lower impulse and desire.

There are always two ways of doing the Yoga – one by the action of a vigilant mind and vital seeing, observing, thinking and deciding what is or is not to be done. Of course, it acts with the Divine Force behind it, drawing or calling in that Force – for otherwise nothing much can be done. But still it is the personal effort that is prominent and assumes most of the burden.

The other way is that of the psychic being, the consciousness opening to the Divine, not only opening the psychic and bringing it forward, but opening the mind, the vital and the physical, receiving the Light, perceiving what is to be done, feeling and seeing it done by the Divine

Force itself and helping constantly by its own vigilant and conscious assent to and call for the Divine working.

Usually there cannot but be a mixture of these two ways until the consciousness is ready to be entirely open, entirely submitted to the Divine's origination of all its action. It is then that all responsibility disappears and there is no personal burden on the shoulders of the sadhak.

*

Whether by tapasya or surrender does not matter, the one thing is to be firm in setting one's face to the goal. Once one has set one's feet on the way, how can one draw back from it to something inferior? If one keeps firm, falls do not matter, one rises up again and goes forward. If one is firm towards the goal, there can be on the way to the Divine no eventual failure. And if there is something within you that drives, as surely there is, falterings or falls or failure of faith make no eventual difference. One has to go on till the struggle is over and there is the straight and open and thornless way before us.

*

The fire is the divine fire of aspiration and inner tapasya. When the fire descends again and again with increasing force and magnitude into the darkness of human ignorance, it at first seems swallowed up and absorbed in the darkness, but more and more of the descent changes the darkness into light, the ignorance and unconsciousness of the human mind into spiritual consciousness.

*

To practise Yoga implies the will to overcome all attachments and turn to the Divine alone. The principal thing in the Yoga is to trust in the Divine Grace at every step, to direct the thought continually to the Divine and to offer oneself till the being opens and the Mother's force can be felt working in the Adhar.

*

In this Yoga the whole principle is to open oneself to the Divine Influence. It is there above you and, if you can once become conscious of it, you have then to call it down into you. It descends into the mind and into the body as Peace, as a Light, as a Force that works, as the Presence of the Divine with or without form, as Ananda. Before one has this consciousness, one has to have faith and aspire for the opening. Aspiration, call, prayer are forms of one and the same thing and are all effective; you can take the form that comes to you or is easiest to you. The other way is concentration; you concentrate your consciousness in the heart (some do it in the head or above the head) and meditate on the Mother in the heart and call her in there. One can do either and both at different times – whatever comes naturally to you or you are moved to do at the moment. Especially in the beginning the one great necessity is to get the mind quiet, reject at the time of meditation all thoughts and movements that are foreign to the sadhana. In the quiet mind there will be a progressive preparation for the experience. But you must not become impatient, if all is not done at once; it takes time to bring entire quiet into the mind; you have to go on till the consciousness is ready.

*

In the practice of Yoga, what you aim at can only come by the opening of the being to the Mother's force and the persistent rejection of all egoism and demand and desire, all motives except the aspiration for the Divine Truth. If this is rightly done, the Divine Power and Light will begin to work and bring in the peace and equanimity, the inner strength, the purified devotion and the increasing consciousness and self-knowledge which are the necessary foundation for the siddhi of the Yoga.

*

The Truth for you is to feel the Divine in you, open to the Mother and work for the Divine till you are aware of her in all your activities. There must be the consciousness of the divine presence in your heart and the divine guidance in your acts. This the psychic being can easily, swiftly, deeply feel if it is fully awake; once the psychic has felt it, it can spread to the mental and vital also.

*

The only truth in your other experience – which, you say, seems at the time so true to you, – is that it is hopeless for you or anyone to get out of the inferior consciousness by your or his unaided effort. That is why when you sink into this inferior consciousness, everything seems hopeless to you, because you lose hold for a time of the true consciousness. But the suggestion is untrue, because you have an opening to the Divine and are not bound to remain in the inferior consciousness.

When you are in the true consciousness, then you see that everything can be done, even if at present only a slight beginning has been made; but a beginning is enough, once the Force, the Power are there. For the truth is that it can do everything and only time and the soul's aspiration are needed for the entire change and the soul's fulfilment.

*

The conditions for following the Mother's Will are to turn to her for Light and Truth and Strength, to aspire that no other force shall influence or lead you, to make no demands or conditions in the vital, to keep a quiet mind ready to receive the Truth but not insisting on its own ideas and formations, – finally to keep the psychic awake and in front, so that you may be in a constant contact and know truly what her will is; for the mind and vital can mistake other impulsions and suggestions for the Divine Will, but the psychic once awakened makes no mistake.

A perfect perfection in working is only possible after supramentalisation; but a relative good working is possible on the lower planes, if one is in contact with the Divine and careful, vigilant and conscious in mind and vital and body. That is a condition, besides, which is preparatory and almost indispensable for the supreme liberation.

*

One who fears monotony and wants something new would not be able to do Yoga or at least this Yoga which needs an inexhaustible perseverance and patience. The fear of death shows a vital weakness which is also contrary to a capacity for Yoga. Equally, one who is under the

domination of his passions, would find the Yoga difficult
and, unless supported by a true inner call and a sincere
and strong aspiration for the spiritual consciousness and
union with the Divine, might very easily fall fatally and his
effort come to nothing.

*

As for working, it depends on what you mean by the
word. Desire often leads either to excess of effort, meaning often much labour and a limited fruit, with strain,
exhaustion and in case of difficulty or failure, despon-
dence, disbelief or revolt; or else it leads to pulling down
the force. That can be done, but except for the yogically
strong and experienced, it is not always safe, though it
may be often very effective; not safe, first, because it may
lead to violent reactions or it brings down contrary or
wrong or mixed forces which the sadhak is not experienced
enough to distinguish from the true ones. Or else it may
substitute the sadhak's own limited power of experience
or his mental and vital constructions for the free gift and
true leading of the Divine. Cases differ, each has his own
way of sadhana. But for you what I would recommend is
constant openness, a quiet steady aspiration, no over-
eagerness, a cheerful trust and patience.

*

It is very unwise for anyone to claim prematurely to
have possession of the supermind or even to have a taste
of it. The claim is usually accompanied by an outburst of
super-egoism, some radical blunder of perception or a
gross fall, wrong condition and wrong movement. A certain

spiritual humility, a serious unarrogant look at oneself and quiet perception of the imperfections of one's present nature and, instead of self-esteem and self-assertion, a sense of the necessity of exceeding one's present self, not from egoistic ambition, but from an urge towards the Divine would be, it seems to me, for this frail, terrestrial and human composition far better conditions for proceeding towards the supramental change.

*

It is the psychic surrender in the physical that you have begun to experience.

All the parts are essentially offered, but the surrender has to be made complete by the growth of the psychic self-offering in all of them and in all their movements separately and together.

To be enjoyed by the Divine is to be entirely surrendered so that one feels the Divine Presence, Power, Light, Ananda possessing the whole being rather than oneself possessing these things for one's own satisfaction. It is a much greater ecstasy to be thus surrendered and possessed by the Divine than oneself to be the possessor. At the same time by this surrender there comes also a calm and happy mastery of self and nature.

*

Get the psychic being in front and keep it there, putting its power on the mind, vital and physical, so that it shall communicate to them its force of single-minded aspiration, trust, faith, surrender, direct and immediate detection of whatever is wrong in the nature and turned towards ego and error, away from Light and Truth.

Eliminate egoism in all its forms; eliminate it from every movement of your consciousness.

Develop the cosmic consciousness – let the egocentric outlook disappear in wideness, impersonality, the sense of the Cosmic Divine, the perception of universal forces, the realisation and understanding of the cosmic manifestation, the play.

Find in place of ego the true being – a portion of the Divine, issued from the World-Mother and an instrument of the manifestation. This sense of being a portion of the Divine and an instrument should be free from all pride, sense or claim of ego or assertion of superiority, demand or desire. For if these elements are there, then it is not the true thing.

Most in doing Yoga live in the mind, vital, physical, lit up occasionally or to some extent by the Higher Mind and by the Illumined Mind; but to prepare for the supramental change it is necessary (as soon as, personally, the time has come) to open up to the Intuition and the Overmind, so that these may make the whole being and the whole nature ready for the supramental change. Allow the consciousness quietly to develop and widen and the knowledge of these things will progressively come.

Calm, discrimination, detachment (but not indifference) are all very important, for their opposites impede very much the transforming action. Intensity of aspiration should be there, but it must go along with these. No hurry, no inertia, neither rajasic over-eagerness nor tamasic discouragement – a steady and persistent but quiet call and working. No snatching or clutching at realisation, but allowing realisation to come from within and above and observing accurately its field, its nature, its limits.

Let the power of the Mother work in you, but be careful to avoid any mixture or substitution, in its place, of either a magnified ego-working or a force of Ignorance presenting itself as Truth. Aspire especially for the elimination of all obscurity and unconsciousness in the nature.

These are the main conditions of preparation for the supramental change; but none of them is easy, and they must be complete before the nature can be said to be ready. If the true attitude (psychic, unegoistic, open only to the Divine Force) can be established, then the process can go on much more quickly. To take and keep the true attitude, to further the change in oneself, is the help that can be given, the one thing asked to assist the general change.

III

IN DIFFICULTY

There are always difficulties and a hampered progress in the early stages and a delay in the opening of the inner doors until the being is ready. If you feel whenever you meditate the quiescence and the flashes of the inner Light and if the inward urge is growing so strong that the external hold is decreasing and the vital disturbances are losing their force, that is already a great progress. The road of Yoga is long, every inch of ground has to be won against much resistance and no quality is more needed by the sadhak than patience and single-minded perseverance with a faith that remains firm through all difficulties, delays and apparent failures.

*

These obstacles are usual in the first stages of the sadhana. They are due to the nature being not yet sufficiently receptive. You should find out where the obstacle is, in the mind or the vital, and try to widen the consciousness there, call in more purity and peace and in that purity and peace offer that part of your being sincerely and wholly to the Divine Power.

*

Each part of the nature wants to go on with its old movements and refuses, so far as it can, to admit a radical change and progress, because that would subject it to something higher than itself and deprive it of its sovereignty in its own field, its separate empire. It is this that makes transformation so long and difficult a process.

Mind gets dulled because at its lower basis is the physical mind with its principle of tamas or inertia – for in matter inertia is the fundamental principle. A constant or long continuity of higher experiences produces in this part of mind a sense of exhaustion or reaction of unease or dullness. Trance or *samādhi* is a way of escape – the body is made quiet, the physical mind is in a state of torpor, the inner consciousness is left free to go on with its experiences. The disadvantage is that trance becomes indispensable and the problem of the waking consciousness is not solved; it remains imperfect.

*

If the difficulty in meditation is that thoughts of all kinds come in, that is not due to hostile forces but to the ordinary nature of the human mind. All sadhaks have this difficulty and with many it lasts for a very long time. There are several ways of getting rid of it. One of them is to look at the thoughts and observe what is the nature of the human mind as they show it but not to give any sanction and to let them run down till they come to a standstill – this is a way recommended by Vivekananda in his Raja-yoga. Another is to look at the thoughts as not one's own, to stand back as the witness Purusha and refuse the sanction – the thoughts are regarded as things coming from outside, from Prakriti, and they must be felt as if they were passers-by crossing the mind-space with whom one has no connection and in whom one takes no interest. In this way it usually happens that after a time the mind divides into two, a part which is the mental witness watch-

ing and perfectly undisturbed and quiet and a part which is
the object of observation, the Prakriti part in which the
thoughts cross or wander. Afterwards one can proceed to
silence or quiet the Prakriti part also. There is a third, an
active method by which one looks to see where the
thoughts come from and finds they come not from oneself,
but from outside the head as it were; if one can detect
them coming, then, before they enter, they have to be
thrown away altogether. This is perhaps the most difficult
way and not all can do it, but if it can be done it is the
shortest and most powerful road to silence.

*

It is necessary to observe and know the wrong movements in you; for they are the source of your trouble and
have to be persistently rejected if you are to be free.

But do not be always thinking of your defects and
wrong movements. Concentrate more upon what you are
to be, on the ideal with the faith that, since it is the goal
before you, it must and will come.

To be always observing faults and wrong movements
brings depression and discourages the faith. Turn your
eyes more to the coming light and less to any immediate
darkness. Faith, cheerfulness, confidence in the ultimate
victory are the things that help, – they make the progress
easier and swifter.

Make more of the good experiences that come to you;
one experience of the kind is more important than the
lapses and failures. When it ceases, do not repine or allow
yourself to be discouraged, but be quiet within and aspire
for its renewal in a stronger form leading to still deeper
and fuller experience.

Aspire always, but with more quietude, opening your-self to the Divine simply and wholly.

*

The lower vital in most human beings is full of grave defects and of movements that respond to hostile forces. A constant psychic opening, a persistent rejection of these influences, a separation of oneself from all hostile sugges-tions and the inflow of the calm, light, peace, purity of the Mother's power would eventually free the system from the siege.

What is needed is to be quiet and more and more quiet, to look on these influences as something not yourself which has intruded, to separate yourself from it and deny it and to abide in a quiet confidence in the Divine Power. If your psychic being asks for the Divine and your mind is sincere and calls for liberation from the lower nature and from all hostile forces and if you can call the Mother's power into your heart and rely upon it more than on your own strength, this siege will in the end be driven away from you and strength and peace take its place.

*

The lower nature is ignorant and undivine, not in itself hostile but shut to the Light and Truth. The hostile forces are antidivine, not merely undivine; they make use of the lower nature, pervert it, fill it with distorted movements and by that means influence man and even try to enter and possess or at least entirely control him.

Free yourself from all exaggerated self-depreciation and the habit of getting depressed by the sense of sin, difficulty or failure. These feelings do not really help, on the contrary, they are an immense obstacle and hamper the progress. They belong to the religious, not to the Yogic mentality. The Yogin should look on all the defects of the nature as movements of the lower Prakriti common to all and reject them calmly, firmly and persistently with full confidence in the Divine Power – without weakness or depression or negligence and without excitement, impatience or violence.

*

The rule in Yoga is not to let the depression depress you, to stand back from it, observe its cause and remove the cause; for the cause is always in oneself, perhaps a vital defect somewhere, a wrong movement indulged or a petty desire causing a recoil, sometimes by its satisfaction, sometimes by its disappointment. In Yoga a desire satisfied, a false movement given its head produces very often a worse recoil than disappointed desire.

What is needed for you is to live more deeply within, less in the outer vital and mental part which is exposed to these touches. The inmost psychic being is not oppressed by them; it stands in its own closeness to the Divine and sees the small surface movements as surface things foreign to the true Being.

*

In your dealing with your difficulties and the wrong movements that assail you, you are probably making the mistake of identifying yourself with them too much and regarding them as part of your own nature. You should

rather draw back from them, detach and dissociate yourself from them, regard them as movements of the universal lower imperfect and impure Nature, forces that
enter into you and try to make you their instrument for
their self-expression. By so detaching and dissociating
yourself it will be more possible for you to discover and to
live more and more in a part of yourself, your inner or
your psychic being which is not attacked or troubled by
these movements, finds them foreign to itself and automatically refuses assent to them and feels itself always
turned to or in contact with the Divine Forces and the
higher planes of consciousness. Find that part of your
being and live in it; to be able to do so is the true foundation of the Yoga.

By so standing back it will be easier also for you to find
a quiet poise in yourself, behind the surface struggle, from
which you can more effectively call in the help to deliver
you. The Divine presence, calm, peace, purity, force,
light, joy, wideness are above waiting to descend in you.
Find this quietude behind and your mind also will become
quieter and through the quiet mind you can call down the
descent first of the purity and peace and then of the Divine
Force. If you can feel this peace and purity descending
into you, you can then call it down again and again till it
begins to settle; you will feel too the Force working in you
to change the movements and transform the consciousness. In this working you will be aware of the presence
and power of the Mother. Once that is done, all the rest
will be a question of time and of the progressive evolution
in you of your true and divine nature.

*

The existence of imperfections, even many and serious imperfections, cannot be a *permanent* bar to progress in the Yoga. (I do not speak of a recovery of the former opening, for according to my experience, what comes after a period of obstruction or struggle is usually a new and wider opening, some larger consciousness and an advance on what had been gained before and seems – but only seems – to be lost for the moment.) The only bar that can be permanent – but need not be, for this too can change – is insincerity, and this does not exist in you. If imperfection were a bar, then no man could succeed in Yoga; for all are imperfect, and I am not sure, from what I have seen, that it is not those who have the greatest power for Yoga who have too, very often, or have had the greatest imperfections. You know, I suppose, the comment of Socrates on his own character; that could be said by many great Yogins of their own initial human nature. In Yoga the one thing that counts in the end is sincerity and with it the patience to persist in the path – many even without this patience go through, for in spite of revolt, impatience, depression, despondency, fatigue, temporary loss of faith, a force greater than one's outer self, the force of the Spirit, the drive of the soul's need, pushes them through the cloud and the mist to the goal before them. Imperfections can be stumbling-blocks and give one a bad fall for the moment, but not a permanent bar. Obstructions due to some resistance in the nature can be more serious causes of delay, but they too do not last for ever.

The length of your period of dullness is also no sufficient reason for losing belief in your capacity or your spiritual destiny. I believe that alternations of bright and dark periods are almost a universal experience of Yogis, and the exceptions are very rare. If one inquires into the

reason of this phenomenon, – very unpleasant to our
impatient human nature, – it will be found, I think, that
they are in the main two. The first is that the human
consciousness either cannot bear a constant descent of the
Light or Power or Ananda, or cannot at once receive and
absorb it; it needs periods of assimilation; but this assimilation goes on behind the veil of the surface consciousness; the experience or the realisation that has descended
retires behind the veil and leaves this outer or surface
consciousness to lie fallow and become ready for a new
descent. In the more developed stages of the Yoga these
dark or dull periods become shorter, less trying as well as
uplifted by the sense of the greater consciousness which,
though not acting for immediate progress, yet remains and
sustains the outer nature. The second cause is some resistance, something in the human nature that has not felt the
former descent, is not ready, is perhaps unwilling to
change, – often it is some strong habitual formation of the
mind or the vital or some temporary inertia of the physical
consciousness and not exactly a part of the nature, – and
this, whether showing or concealing itself, thrusts up the
obstacle. If one can detect the cause in oneself, acknow-
ledge it, see its workings and call down the Power for its
removal, then the periods of obscurity can be greatly
shortened and their acuity becomes less. But in any case
the Divine Power is working always behind and one day,
perhaps when one least expects it, the obstacle breaks, the
clouds vanish and there is again the light and the sunshine.
The best thing in these cases is, if one can manage it, not
to fret, not to despond, but to insist quietly and keep
oneself open, spread to the Light and waiting in faith for it
to come; that I have found shortens these ordeals. Afterwards, when the obstacle disappears, one finds that a

great progress has been made and that the consciousness is far more capable of receiving and retaining than before. There is a return for all the trials and ordeals of the spiritual life.

*

While the recognition of the Divine Power and the attunement of one's own nature to it cannot be done without the recognition of the imperfections in that nature, yet it is a wrong attitude to put too much stress either on them or on the difficulties they create, or to distrust the Divine working because of the difficulties one experiences, or to lay too continual an emphasis on the dark side of things. To do this increases the force of the difficulties, gives a greater right of continuance to the imperfections. I do not insist on a Coueistic optimism – although excessive optimism is more helpful than excessive pessimism; that (Coueism) tends to cover up difficulties and there is, besides, always a measure to be observed in things. But there is no danger of your covering them up and deluding yourself with too bright an outlook; quite the contrary, you always lay stress too much on the shadows and by so doing thicken them and obstruct your outlets of escape into the Light. Faith, more faith! Faith in your possibilities, faith in the Power that is at work behind the veil, faith in the work that is to be done and the offered guidance.

There cannot be any high endeavour, least of all in the spiritual field, which does not raise or encounter grave obstacles of a very persistent character. These are both internal and external, and, although in the large they are fundamentally the same for all, there may be a great

difference in the distribution of their stress or the outward
form they take. But the one real difficulty is the attunement of the nature with the working of the Divine Light
and Power. Get that solved and the others will either
disappear or take a subordinate place; and even with
those difficulties that are of a more general character,
more lasting because they are inherent in the work of
transformation, they will not weigh so heavily because the
sense of the supporting Force and a greater power to
follow its movement will be there.

*

The entire oblivion of the experience means merely that
there is still no sufficient bridge between the inner consciousness which has the experience in a kind of samadhi
and the exterior waking consciousness. It is when the
higher consciousness has made the bridge between them
that the outer also begins to remember.

*

These fluctuations in the force of the aspiration and the
power of the sadhana are unavoidable and common to all
sadhaks until the whole being has been made ready for the
transformation. When the psychic is in front or active and
the mind and vital consent, then there is the intensity.
When the psychic is less prominent and the lower vital has
its ordinary movements or the mind its ignorant action,
then the opposing forces can come in unless the sadhak is
very vigilant. Inertia comes usually from the ordinary
physical consciousness, especially when the vital is not
actively supporting the sadhana. These things can only be

cured by a persistent bringing down of the higher spiritual consciousness into all the parts of the being.

*

An occasional sinking of the consciousness happens to everybody. The causes are various, some touch from outside, something not yet changed or not sufficiently changed in the vital, especially the lower vital, some inertia or obscurity rising up from the physical parts of nature. When it comes, remain quiet, open yourself to the Mother and call back the true conditions and aspire for a clear and undisturbed discrimination showing you from within yourself the cause of the thing that needs to be set right.

*

There are always pauses of preparation and assimilation between two movements. You must not regard these with fretfulness or impatience as if they were untoward gaps in the sadhana. Besides, the Force rises up lifting part of the nature on a higher level and then comes down to a lower layer to raise it; this motion of ascent and descent is often extremely trying because the mind partial to an ascent in a straight line and the vital eager for rapid fulfilment cannot understand or follow the intricate movement and are apt to be distressed by it or resent it. But the transformation of the whole nature is not an easy thing to accomplish and the Force that does it knows better than our mental ignorance or our vital impatience.

*

It is a very serious difficulty in one's Yoga – the absence of a central will always superior to the waves of the Prakriti forces, always in touch with the Mother, imposing its central aim and aspiration on the nature. That is because you have not yet learned to live in your central being; you have been accustomed to run with every wave of Force, no matter of what kind, that rushed upon you and to identify yourself with it for the time being. It is one of the things that has to be unlearned; you must find your central being with the psychic as its basis and live in it.

*

However hard the fight, the only thing is to fight it out now and here to the end.

The trouble is that you have never fully faced and conquered the real obstacle. There is in a very fundamental part of your nature a strong formation of ego-individuality which has mixed in your spiritual aspiration a clinging element of pride and spiritual ambition. This formation has never consented to be broken up in order to give place to something more true and divine. Therefore, when the Mother has put her force upon you or when you yourself have pulled the force upon you, this in you has always prevented it from doing its work in its own way. It has begun itself building according to the ideas of the mind or some demand of the ego, trying to make its own creation in its "own way", by its own strength, its own sadhana, its own tapasya. There has never been here any real surrender, any giving up of yourself freely and simply into the hands of the Divine Mother. And yet that is the only way to succeed in the supramental Yoga. To be a Yogi, a Sannyasi, a Tapaswi is not the object here. The object is transformation, and the transformation can only be done by a force infinitely greater than your own; it can only be done by being truly like a child in the hands of the Divine Mother.

*

There is no reason why you should abandon hope of success in the Yoga. The state of depression which you now feel is temporary and it comes even upon the strongest sadhaks at one time or another or even often recurs. The only thing needed is to hold firm with the awakened part of the being, to reject all contrary suggestions and to wait, opening yourself as much as you can to the true Power, till the crisis or change of which this depression is a stage is completed. The suggestions which come to your mind telling you that you are not fit and that you must go back to the ordinary life are promptings from a hostile source. Ideas of this kind must always be rejected as inventions of the lower nature; even if they are founded on appearances which seem convincing to the ignorant mind, they are false, because they exaggerate a passing movement and represent it as the decisive and definite truth. There is only one truth in you on which you have to lay constant hold, the truth of your divine possibilities and the call of the higher Light to your nature. If you hold to that always, or, even if you are momentarily shaken from your hold, return constantly to it, it will justify itself in the end in spite of all difficulties and obstacles and stumblings. All that resists will disappear in time with the progressive unfolding of your spiritual nature.

What is needed is the conversion and surrender of the vital part. It must learn to demand only the highest truth

and to forego all insistence on the satisfaction of its inferior impulses and desires. It is this adhesion of the vital
being that brings the full satisfaction and joy of the whole
nature in the spiritual life. When that is there, it will be
impossible even to think of returning to the ordinary
existence. Meanwhile the mental will and the psychic aspiration must be your support; if you insist, the vital will
finally yield and be converted and surrender.

Fix upon your mind and heart the resolution to live for
the Divine Truth and for that alone; reject all that is
contrary and incompatible with it and turn away from the
lower desires; aspire to open yourself to the Divine Power
and to no other. Do this in all sincerity and the present
and living help you need will not fail you.

*

The attitude you have taken is the right one. It is this
feeling and attitude which help you to overcome so rapidly
the attacks that sometimes fall upon you and throw you
out of the right consciousness. As you say, difficulties so
taken become opportunities; the difficulty faced in the
right spirit and conquered, one finds that an obstacle has
disappeared, a first step forward has been taken. To question, to resist in some part of the being increases trouble
and difficulties – that is why an unquestioning acceptance,
an unfailing obedience to the directions of the Guru was
laid down as indispensable in the old Indian Yogas – it was
demanded not for the sake of the Guru, but for the sake of
the Shishya.

*

It is one thing to see things and quite another to let them enter into you. One has to experience many things, to see and observe, to bring them into the field of the consciousness and know what they are. But there is no reason why you should allow them to enter into you and possess you. It is only the Divine or what comes from the Divine that can be admitted to enter you.

To say that all light is good is as if you said that all water is good – or even that all clear or transparent water is good: it would not be true. One must see what is the nature of the light or where it comes from or what is in it, before one can say that it is the true Light. False lights exist and misleading lustres, lower lights too that belong to the being's inferior reaches. One must therefore be on one's guard and distinguish; the true discrimination has to come by growth of the psychic feeling and a purified mind and experience.

*

The cry you heard was not in the physical heart, but in the emotional centre. The breaking of the wall meant the breaking of the obstacle or at least of some obstacle there between your inner and your outer being. Most people live in their ordinary outer ignorant personality which does not easily open to the Divine; but there is an inner being within them of which they do not know, which can easily open to the Truth and the Light. But there is a wall which divides them from it, a wall of obscurity and unconsciousness. When it breaks down, then there is a release; the feelings of calm, Ananda, joy which you had immediately afterwards were due to that release. The cry you heard was the cry of the vital part in you overcome by the suddenness of the breaking of the wall and the opening.

*

The consciousness is usually imprisoned in the body, centralised in the brain and heart and navel centres (mental, emotional, sensational); when you feel it or something of it go up and take its station above the head, that is the liberation of the imprisoned consciousness from the body-formula. It is the mental in you that goes up there, gets into touch with something higher than the ordinary mind and from there puts the higher mental will on the rest for transformation. The trembling and the heat come from a resistance, an absence of habituation in the body and the vital to this demand and to this liberation. When the mental consciousness can take its stand permanently or at will above like this, then this first liberation becomes accomplished (*siddha*). From there the mental being can open freely to the higher planes or to the cosmic existence and its forces and can also act with greater liberty and power on the lower nature.

*

The method of the Divine Manifestation is through calm and harmony, not through a catastrophic upheaval. The latter is the sign of a struggle, generally of conflicting vital forces, but at any rate a struggle on the inferior plane.

You think too much of the adverse forces. That kind of preoccupation causes much unnecessary struggle. Fix your mind on the positive side. Open to the Mother's power, concentrate on her protection, call for light, calm and peace and purity and growth into the divine consciousness and knowledge.

The idea of tests also is not a healthy idea and ought not to be pushed too far. Tests are applied not by the Divine but by the forces of the lower planes – mental, vital, physical – and allowed by the Divine because that is part of the soul's training and helps it to know itself, its powers and the limitations it has to outgrow. The Mother is not testing you at every moment, but rather helping you at every moment to rise beyond the necessity of tests and difficulties which belong to the inferior consciousness. To be always conscious of that help will be your best safe-guard against all attacks whether of adverse powers or of your own lower nature.

*

The hostile forces have a certain self-chosen function: it is to test the condition of the individual, of the work, of the earth itself and their readiness for the spiritual descent and fulfilment. At every step of the journey, they are there attacking furiously, criticising, suggesting, imposing despondency or inciting to revolt, raising unbelief, amas-sing difficulties. No doubt, they put a very exaggerated interpretation on the rights given them by their function, making mountains even out of what seems to us a mole-hill. A little trifling false step or mistake and they appear on the road and clap a whole Himalaya as a barrier across it. But this opposition has been permitted from of old not merely as a test or ordeal, but as a compulsion on us to seek a greater strength, a more perfect self-knowledge, an intenser purity and force of aspiraton, a faith that nothing can crush, a more powerful descent of the Divine Grace.

*

The Power does not descend with the object of raising up the lower forces, but in the way it has to work at present, that uprising comes in as a reaction to the working. What is needed is the establishment of the calm and wide consciousness at the base of the whole Nature, so that when the lower nature appears it will not be as an attack or struggle but as if a Master of forces were there seeing the defects of the present machinery and doing step by step what is necessary to remedy and change it.

*

It is the forces of the Ignorance that begin first to lay siege from outside and then make a mass attack in order to overpower and capture. Every time such an attack can be defeated and cast out, there is a clearance in the being, a new field gained for the Mother in the mind, vital or physical or the adjacent parts of the nature. That the place in the vital occupied by the Mother is increasing is shown by the fact that you are now offering a stronger resistance to these sieges that used formerly to overpower you altogether.

To be able to call the Mother's presence or force at such times is the best way to meet the difficulty.

It is with the Mother who is always with you and in you that you converse. The only thing is to hear aright, so that no other voice can ape hers or come in between her and you.

*

Your mind and psychic being are concentrated on the spiritual aim and open to the Divine – that is why the Influence comes down only to the head and as far as the heart. But the vital being and nature and physical consciousness are under the influence of the lower nature. As long as the vital and physical being are not surrendered or do not on their own account call for the higher life, the struggle is likely to continue.

Surrender everything, reject all other desires or interests, call on the Divine Shakti to open the vital nature and bring down calm, peace, light, Ananda into all the centres. Aspire, await with faith and patience the result. All depends on a complete sincerity and an integral consecration and aspiration.

The world will trouble you so long as any part of you belongs to the world. It is only if you belong entirely to the Divine that you can become free.

*

One who has not the courage to face patiently and firmly life and its difficulties will never be able to go through the still greater inner difficulties of the sadhana. The very first lesson in this Yoga is to face life and its trials with a quiet mind, a firm courage and an entire reliance on the Divine Shakti.

*

Suicide is an absurd solution; he is quite mistaken in thinking that it will give him peace. He will only carry his difficulties with him into a more miserable condition of existence beyond and bring them back to another life on

earth. The only remedy is to shake off these morbid ideas
and face life with a clear will for some definite work to be
done as the life's aim and with a quiet and active courage.

* * * * *

Sadhana has to be done in the body, it cannot be done
by the soul without the body. When the body drops, the
soul goes wandering in other worlds – and finally it comes
back to another life and another body. Then all the difficulties it had not solved meet it again in the new life. So
what is the use of leaving the body?

Moreover, if one throws away the body wilfully, one
suffers much in the other worlds and when one is born
again, it is in worse, not in better conditions.

The only sensible thing is to face the difficulties in this
life and this body and conquer them.

*

The goal of Yoga is always hard to reach, but this one is
more difficult than any other, and it is only for those who
have the call, the capacity, the willingness to face everything and every risk, even the risk of failure, and the will
to progress towards an entire selflessness, desirelessness
and surrender.

*

Let nothing and nobody come between you and the
Mother's force. It is on your admitting and keeping that
force and responding to the true inspiration and not on
any ideas the mind may form that success will depend.

Even ideas or plans which might otherwise be useful, will fail if there is not behind them the true spirit and the true force and influence.

*

The difficulty must have come from distrust and disobedience. For distrust and disobedience are like falsehood (they are themselves a falsity, based on false ideas and impulses), they interfere in the action of the Power, prevent it from being felt or from working fully and diminish the force of the Protection.

Not only in your inward concentration, but in your outward acts and movements you must take the right attitude. If you do that and put everything under the Mother's guidance, you will find that difficulties begin to diminish or are much more easily got over and things become steadily smoother.

In your work and acts you must do the same as in your concentration. Open to the Mother, put them under her guidance, call in the peace, the supporting Power, the protection and, in order that they may work, reject all wrong influences that might come in their way by creating wrong, careless or unconscious movements.

Follow this principle and your whole being will become one, under one rule, in the peace and sheltering Power and Light.

*

When I spoke of being faithful to the light of the soul and the divine Call, I was not referring to anything in the past or to any lapse on your part. I was simply affirming

the great need in all crises and attacks, – to refuse to listen
to any suggestions, impulses, lures and to oppose to them
all the call of the Truth, the imperative beckoning of the
Light. In all doubt and depression, to say, "I belong to the
Divine, I cannot fail"; to all suggestions of impurity and
unfitness, to reply, "I am a child of Immortality chosen by
the Divine; I have but to be true to myself and to Him –
the victory is sure; even if I fell, I would rise again"; to all
impulses to depart and serve some smaller ideal, to reply,
"This is the greatest, this is the Truth that alone can satisfy
the soul within me; I will endure through all tests and
tribulations to the very end of the divine journey." This is
what I mean by faithfulness to the Light and the Call.

IV

DESIRE – FOOD – SEX

All the ordinary vital movements are foreign to the true being and come from outside; they do not belong to the soul nor do they originate in it but are waves from the general Nature, Prakriti.

The desires come from outside, enter the subconscious vital and rise to the surface. It is only when they rise to the surface and the mind becomes aware of them, that we become conscious of the desire. It seems to us to be our own because we feel it thus rising from the vital into the mind and do not know that it came from outside. What belongs to the vital, to the being, what makes it responsible is not the desire itself, but the habit of responding to the waves or the currents of suggestion that come into it from the universal Prakriti.

*

The rejection of desire is essentially the rejection of the element of craving, putting that out from the consciousness itself as a foreign element not belonging to the true self and the inner nature. But refusal to indulge the suggestions of desire is also a part of the rejection; to abstain from the action suggested, if it is not the right action, must be included in the Yogic discipline. It is only when this is done in the wrong way, by a mental ascetic principle or a hard moral rule, that it can be called suppression. The difference between suppression and an inward essential rejection is the difference between mental or moral control and a spiritual purification.

When one lives in the true consciousness one feels the desires outside oneself, entering from outside, from the universal lower Prakriti, into the mind and the vital parts. In the ordinary human condition this is not felt; men become aware of the desire only when it is there, when it has come inside and found a lodging or a habitual harbourage and so they think it is their own and a part of themselves. The first condition for getting rid of desire is, therefore, to become conscious with the true consciousness; for then it becomes much easier to dismiss it than when one has to struggle with it as if it were a constituent part of oneself to be thrown out from the being. It is easier to cast off an accretion than to excise what is felt as a parcel of our substance.

When the psychic being is in front, then also to get rid of desire becomes easy; for the psychic being has in itself no desires, it has only aspirations and a seeking and love for the Divine and all things that are or tend towards the Divine. The constant prominence of the psychic being tends of itself to bring out the true consciousness and set right almost automatically the movements of the nature.

*

Demand and desire are only two different aspects of the same thing – nor is it necessary that a feeling should be agitated or restless to be a desire; it can be, on the contrary, quietly fixed and persistent or persistently recurrent. Demand or desire comes from the mental or the vital, but a psychic or spiritual need is a different thing. The psychic does not demand or desire – it aspires; it does not make conditions for its surrender or withdraw if its aspiration is not immediately satisfied – for the psychic has

complete trust in the Divine or in the Guru and can wait
for the right time or the hour of the Divine Grace. The
psychic has an insistence of its own, but it puts its pressure
not on the Divine, but on the nature, placing a finger of
light on all the defects there that stand in the way of the
realisation, sifting out all that is mixed, ignorant or imperfect in the experience or in the movements of the Yoga
and never satisfied with itself or with the nature till it has
got it perfectly open to the Divine, free from all forms of
ego, surrendered, simple and right in the attitude and all
the movements. This is what has to be established entirely
in the mind and vital and in the physical consciousness
before supramentalisation of the whole nature is possible.
Otherwise what one gets is more or less brilliant, half-
luminous, half-cloudy illuminations and experiences on
the mental and vital and physical planes inspired either
from some larger mind or larger vital or at the best from
the mental reaches above the human that intervene between the intellect and the Overmind. These can be very
stimulating and satisfying up to a certain point and are
good for those who want some spiritual realisation on
these planes; but the supramental realisation is something
much more difficult and exacting in its conditions and the
most difficult of all is to bring it down to the physical level.

*

Desire takes a long time to get rid of entirely. But, if
you can once get it out of the nature and realise it as a
force coming from outside and putting its claws into the
vital and physical, it will be easier to get rid of the invader.
You are too accustomed to feel it as part of yourself or
planted in you – that makes it more difficult for you to

deal with its movements and dismiss its ancient control over you.

You should not rely on anything else alone, however helpful it may seem, but chiefly, primarily, fundamentally on the Mother's Force. The Sun and the Light may be a help, and will be if it is the true Light and the true Sun, but cannot take the place of the Mother's Force.

*

The *necessities* of a sadhak should be as few as possible; for there are only a very few things that are real necessities in life. The rest are either utilities or things decorative to life or luxuries. These a Yogin has a right to possess or enjoy only on one of two conditions –

(*i*) If he uses them during his sadhana solely to train himself in possessing things without attachment or desire and learn to use them rightly, in harmony with the Divine Will, with a proper handling, a just organisation, arrangement and measure – or,

(*ii*) if he has already attained a true freedom from desire and attachment and is not in the least moved or affected in any way by loss of withholding or deprival. If he has any greed, desire, demand, claim for possession or enjoyment, any anxiety, grief, anger or vexation when denied or deprived, he is not free in spirit and his use of the things he possesses is contrary to the spirit of sadhana. Even if he is free in spirit, he will not be fit for possession if he has not learned to use things not for himself, but for the Divine Will, as an instrument, with the right knowledge and action in the use, for the proper equipment of a life lived not for oneself but for and in the Divine.

*

Asceticism for its own sake is not the ideal of this Yoga, but self-control in the vital and right order in the material are a very important part of it – and even an ascetic discipline is better for our purpose than a loose absence of true control. Mastery of the material does not mean having plenty and profusely throwing it out or spoiling it as fast as it comes or faster. Mastery implies in it the right and careful utilisation of things and also a self-control in their use.

*

If you want to do Yoga, you must take more and more in all matters, small or great, the Yogic attitude. In our path that attitude is not one of forceful suppression, but of detachment and equality with regard to the objects of desire. Forceful suppression (fasting comes under the head) stands on the same level as free indulgence; in both cases, the desire remains: in the one it is fed by indulgence, in the other it lies latent and exasperated by suppression. It is only when one stands back, separates oneself from the lower vital, refusing to regard its desires and clamours as one's own, and cultivates an entire equality and equanimity in the consciousness with respect to them that the lower vital itself becomes gradually purified and itself also calm and equal. Each wave of desire as it comes must be observed, as quietly and with as much unmoved detachment as you would observe something going on outside you, and must be allowed to pass, rejected from the consciousness, and the true movement, the true consciousness steadily put in its place.

*

It is the attachment to food, the greed and eagerness for it, making it an unduly important thing in the life, that is contrary to the spirit of Yoga. To be aware that something is pleasant to the palate is not wrong; only one must have no desire nor hankering for it, no exultation in getting it, no displeasure or regret at not getting it. One must be calm and equal, not getting upset or dissatisfied when the food is not tasty or not in abundance – eating the fixed amount that is necessary, not less or more. There should be neither eagerness nor repugnance.

To be always thinking about food and troubling the mind is quite the wrong way of getting rid of the food-desire. Put the food element in the right place in the life, in a small corner, and don't concentrate on it but on other things.

*

Do not trouble your mind about food. Take it in the right quantity (neither too much nor too little), without greed or repulsion, as the means given you by the Mother for the maintenance of the body, in the right spirit, offering it to the Divine in you; then it need not create *tamas*.

*

It is no part of this Yoga to suppress taste, *rasa*, altogether. What is to be got rid of is vital desire and attachment, the greed of food, being overjoyed at getting the food you like, sorry and discontented when you do not have it, giving an undue importance to it. Equality is here the test as in so many other matters.

*

The idea of giving up food is a wrong inspiration. You can go on with a small quantity of food, but not without food altogether, except for a comparatively short time. Remember what the Gita says, "Yoga is not for one who eats in excess nor for one who abstains from eating altogether." Vital energy is one thing – of that one can draw a great amount without food and often it increases with fasting; but physical substance, without which life loses its support, is of a different order.

*

Neither neglect this turn of the nature (food-desire) nor make too much of it; it has to be dealt with, purified and mastered but without giving it too much importance. There are two ways of conquering it – one of detachment, learning to regard food as only a physical necessity and the vital satisfaction of the stomach and the palate as a thing of no importance; the other is to be able to take without insistence or seeking any food given and to find in it (whether pronounced good or bad by others) the equal *rasa*, not of the food for its own sake, but of the universal Ananda.

*

It is a mistake to neglect the body and let it waste away; the body is the means of the sadhana and should be maintained in good order. There should be no attachment to it, but no contempt or neglect either of the material part of our nature.

In this Yoga the aim is not only the union with the higher consciousness but the transformation (by its power) of the lower including the physical nature.

It is not necessary to have desire or greed of food in order to eat. The Yogi eats not out of desire, but to maintain the body.

*

It is a fact that by fasting, if the mind and the nerves are solid or the will-force dynamic, one can get for a time into a state of inner energy and receptivity which is alluring to the mind and the usual reactions of hunger, weakness, intestinal disturbance, etc., can be wholly avoided. But the body suffers by diminution and there can easily develop in the vital a morbid overstrained condition due to the inrush of more vital energy than the nervous system can assimilate or co-ordinate. Nervous people should avoid the temptation to fast, it is often accompanied or followed by delusions and a loss of balance. Especially if there is a motive of hunger-strike or that element comes in, fasting becomes perilous, for it is then an indulgence of a vital movement which may easily become a habit injurious and pernicious to the sadhana. Even if all these reactions are avoided, still there is no sufficient utility in fasting, since the higher energy and receptivity ought to come not by artificial or physical means but by intensity of the consciousness and strong will for the sadhana.

*

The transformation to which we aspire is too vast and complex to come at one stroke; it must be allowed to come by stages. The physical change is the last of these stages and is itself a progressive process.

The inner transformation cannot be brought about by physical means either of a positive or a negative nature. On the contrary, the physical change itself can only be brought about by a descent of the greater supramental consciousness into the cells of the body. Till then at least the body and its supporting energies have to be maintained in part by the ordinary means, food, sleep, etc. Food has to be taken in the right spirit, with the right consciousness; sleep has to be gradually transformed into the Yogic repose. A premature and excessive physical austerity, Tapasya, may endanger the process of the sadhana by establishing a disturbance and abnormality of the forces in the different parts of the system. A great energy may pour into the mental and vital parts, but the nerves and the body may be overstrained and lose the strength to support the play of these higher energies. This is the reason why an extreme physical austerity is not included here as a substantive part of the sadhana.

There is no harm in fasting from time to time for a day or two or in reducing the food taken to a small but sufficient modicum; but entire abstinence for a long period is not advisable.

*

The sadhak has to turn away entirely from the invasion of the vital and the physical by the sex-impulse – for, if he does not conquer the sex-impulse there can be no settling in the body of the divine consciousness and the divine Ananda.

*

It is true that the mere suppression or holding down of desire is not enough, not by itself truly effective, but that does not mean that desires are to be indulged; it means that desires have not merely to be suppressed, but to be rejected from the nature. In place of desire there must be a single-minded aspiration towards the Divine.

As for love, the love must be turned singly towards the Divine. What men call by that name is a vital interchange for mutual satisfaction of desire, vital impulse or physical pleasure. There must be nothing of this interchange between sadhaks; for to seek for it or indulge this kind of impulse only leads away from the sadhana.

*

The whole principle of this Yoga is to give oneself entirely to the Divine alone and to nobody and nothing else, and to bring down into ourselves by union with the Divine Mother-Power all the transcendent light, force, wideness, peace, purity, truth-consciousness and Ananda of the supramental Divine. In this Yoga, therefore, there can be no place for vital relations or interchanges with others; any such relation or interchange immediately ties down the soul to the lower consciousness and its lower nature, prevents the true and full union with the Divine and hampers both the ascent to the supramental Truth-consciousness and the descent of the supramental Ishwari Shakti. Still worse would it be if this interchánge took the form of a sexual relation or a sexual enjoyment, even if kept free from any outward act; therefore these things are absolutely forbidden in the sadhana. It goes without saying that any physical act of the kind is not allowed; but also any subtler form is ruled out. It is only after becoming one with the supramental Divine that we can find our true spiritual relations with others in the Divine; in that higher unity this kind of gross lower vital movement can have no place.

To master the sex-impulse, – to become so much master of the sex-centre that the sexual energy would be drawn upwards, not thrown outwards and wasted – it is so indeed that the force in the seed can be turned into a primal physical energy supporting all the others, *retas* into *ojas*. But no error can be more perilous than to accept the immixture of the sexual desire and some kind of subtle satisfaction of it and look on this as a part of the sadhana. It would be the most effective way to head straight towards spiritual downfall and throw into the atmosphere forces that would block the supramental descent, bringing instead the descent of adverse vital powers to disseminate disturbance and disaster. This deviation must be absolutely thrown away, should it try to occur and expunged from the consciousness, if the Truth is to be brought down and the work is to be done.

It is an error too to imagine that, although the physical sexual action is to be abandoned, yet some inward reproduction of it is part of the transformation of the sex-centre. The action of the animal sex-energy in Nature is a device for a particular purpose in the economy of the material creation in the Ignorance. But the vital excitement that accompanies it makes the most favourable opportunity and vibration in the atmosphere for the in-rush of those very vital forces and beings whose whole business is to prevent the descent of the supramental Light. The pleasure attached to it is a degradation and not a true form of the divine Ananda. The true divine Ananda in the physical has a different quality and movement and substance; self-existent in its essence, its manifestation is dependent only on an inner union with the Divine. You have spoken of Divine Love; but Divine Love, when it touches the physical, does not awaken the gross lower vital propensities; indulgence of them would only repel it and make it withdraw again to the heights from which it is already difficult enough to draw it down into the coarseness of the material creation which it alone can transform. Seek the Divine Love through the only gate through which it will consent to enter, the gate of the psychic being, and cast away the lower vital error.

The transformation of the sex-centre and its energy is needed for the physical siddhi; for this is the support in the body of all the mental, vital and physical forces of the nature. It has to be changed into a mass and a movement of intimate Light, creative Power, pure divine Ananda. It is only the bringing down of the supramental Light, Power and Bliss into the centre that can change it. As to the working afterwards, it is the supramental Truth and the creative vision and will of the Divine Mother that will determine it. But it will be a working of the conscious Truth, not of the Darkness and Ignorance to which sexual desire and enjoyment belong; it will be a power of preservation and free desireless radiation of the life-forces and not of their throwing out and waste. Avoid the imagination that the supramental life will be only a heightened satisfaction of the desires of the vital and the body; nothing can be a greater obstacle to the Truth in its descent than this hope of glorification of the animal in the human nature. Mind wants the supramental state to be a confirmation of its own cherished ideas and preconceptions; the vital wants it to be a glorification of its own desires; the physical wants it to be a rich prolongation of its own comforts and pleasures and habits. If it were to be that, it would be only an exaggerated and highly magnified consummation of the animal and the human nature, not a transition from the human into the Divine.

It is dangerous to think of giving up "all barrier of discrimination and defence against what is trying to descend" upon you. Have you thought what this would mean if what is descending is something not in consonance with the divine Truth, perhaps even adverse? An adverse Power would ask no better condition for getting control over the seeker. It is only the Mother's force and the divine Truth that one should admit without barriers. And even there one must keep the power of discernment in order to detect anything false that comes masquerading as the Mother's force and the divine Truth, and keep too the power of rejection that will throw away all mixture.

Keep faith in your spiritual destiny, draw back from error and open more the psychic being to the direct guidance of the Mother's light and power. If the central will is sincere, each recognition of a mistake can become a stepping-stone to a truer movement and a higher progress.

*

I have stated very briefly in my previous letter my position with regard to the sex-impulse and Yoga. I may add here that my conclusion is not founded on any mental opinion or preconceived moral idea, but on probative facts and on observation and experience. I do not deny that so long as one allows a sort of separation between inner experience and outer consciousness, the latter being left as an inferior activity controlled but not transformed, it is quite possible to have spiritual experiences and make

progress without any entire cessation of the sex-activity.
The mind separates itself from the outer vital (life-parts)
and the physical consciousness and lives its own inner life.
But only a few can really do this with any completeness
and the moment one's experiences extend to the life-plane
and the physical, sex can no longer be treated in this way.
It can become at any moment a disturbing, upsetting and
deforming force. I have observed that to an equal extent
with ego (pride, vanity, ambition) and rajasic greeds and
desires it is one of the main causes of the spiritual casual-
ties that have taken place in sadhana. The attempt to treat
it by detachment without complete excision breaks down;
the attempt to sublimate it, favoured by many modern
mystics in Europe, is a most rash and perilous experiment.
For it is when one mixes up sex and spirituality that there
is the greatest havoc. Even the attempt to sublimate it by
turning it towards the Divine as in the Vaishnava *madhura
bhāva* carries in it a serious danger, as the results of a
wrong turn or use in this method so often show. At any
rate in this Yoga which seeks not only the essential experience of the Divine but a transformation of the whole
being and nature, I have found it an absolute necessity of
the sadhana to aim at a complete mastery over the sex-
force: otherwise the vital consciousness remains a turbid
mixture, the turbidity affecting the purity of the spiri-
tualised mind and seriously hindering the upward turn of
the forces of the body. This Yoga demands a full ascen-
sion of the whole lower or ordinary consciousness to join
the spiritual above it and a full descent of the spiritual
(eventually of the supramental) into the mind, life and
body to transform it. The total ascent is impossible so long
as sex-desire blocks the way; the descent is dangerous so
long as sex-desire is powerful in the vital. For at any

moment an unexcised or latent sex-desire may be the
cause of a mixture which throws back the true descent and
uses the energy acquired for other purposes or turns all
the action of the consciousness towards wrong experience,
turbid and delusive. One must, therefore, clear this obstacle out of the way; otherwise there is either no safety or
no free movement towards finality in the sadhana.

The contrary opinion of which you speak may be due to
the idea that sex is a natural part of the human vital-
physical whole, a necessity like food and sleep, and that its
total inhibition may lead to unbalancing and to serious
disorders. It is a fact that sex suppressed in outward action
but indulged in other ways may lead to disorders of the
system and brain troubles. That is the root of the medical
theory which discourages sexual abstinence. But I have
observed that these things happen only when there is
either secret indulgence of a perverse kind replacing the
normal sexual activity or else an indulgence of it in a kind
of subtle vital way by imagination or by an invisible vital
interchange of an occult kind, – I do not think harm ever
occurs when there is a true spiritual effort at mastery and
abstinence. It is now held by many medical men in Europe
that sexual abstinence, *if it is genuine*, is beneficial; for the
element in the *retas* which serves the sexual act is then
changed into its other element which feeds the energies of
the system, mental, vital and physical – and that justifies
the Indian idea of Brahmacharya, the transformation of
retas into *ojas* and the raising of its energies upward so
that they change into a spiritual force.

As for the method of mastery, it cannot be done by
physical abstinence alone – it proceeds by a process of
combined detachment and rejection. The consciousness
stands back from the sex-impulse, feels it as not its own, as

something alien thrown on it by Nature-force to which it refuses assent or identification – each time a certain movement of rejection throws it more and more outward. The mind remains unaffected; after a time the vital being which is the chief support withdraws from it in the same way, finally the physical consciousness no longer supports it. This process continues until even the subconscient can no longer rouse it up in dream and no further movement comes from the outer Nature-force to rekindle this lower fire. This is the course when the sex-propensity sticks obstinately; but there are some who can eliminate it decisively by a swift radical dropping away from the nature. That, however, is more rare.

It has to be said that the total elimination of the sex-impulse is one of the most difficult things in sadhana and one must be prepared for it to take time. But its total disappearance has been achieved and a practical liberation crossed only by occasional dream-movements from the subconscient is fairly common.

*

As to sexual impulse. Regard it not as something sinful and horrible and attractive at the same time, but as a mistake and wrong movement of the lower nature. Reject it entirely, not by struggling with it, but by drawing back from it, detaching yourself and refusing your consent; look at it as something not your own, but imposed on you by a force of Nature outside you. Refuse all consent to the imposition. If anything in your vital consents, insist on that part of you withdrawing its consent. Call in the Divine Force to help you in your withdrawal and refusal. If you can do this quietly and resolutely and patiently, in the

end your inner will will prevail against the habit of the
outer Nature.

*

There is no reason to be depressed to this extent or to
have these imaginations about failure in the Yoga. It is not
at all a sign that you are unfit for the Yoga. It simply
means that the sexual impulse rejected by the conscious
parts has taken refuge in the subconscient, somewhere
probably in the lower vital-physical and the most physical consciousness where there are some regions not
yet open to the aspiration and the light. The persistence
in sleep of things rejected in the waking consciousness is
a quite common occurrence in the course of the sadhana.

The remedy is:

(i) to get the higher consciousness, its light and the
workings of its power down into the obscurer parts of the
nature,

(ii) to become progressively more conscious in sleep,
with an inner consciousness which is aware of the working
of the sadhana in sleep as in waking,

(iii) to bring to bear the waking will and aspiration on
the body in sleep.

One way to do the last is to make a strong and conscious
suggestion to the body, before sleeping, that the thing
should not happen; the more concrete and physical the
suggestion can be made and the more directly on the
sexual centre, the better. The effect may not be quite
immediate at first or invariable; but usually this kind of
suggestion, if you know how to make it, prevails in the
end: even when it does not prevent the dream, it very

often awakes the consciousness within in time to prevent
untoward consequences.

It is a mistake to allow yourself to be depressed in the
sadhana even by repeated failures. One must be calm,
persistent and more obstinate than the resistance.

*

The trouble of the sex-impulse is bound to dwindle
away if you are in earnest about getting rid of it. The
difficulty is that part of your nature (especially, the lower
vital and the subconscient which is active in sleep) keeps
the memory and attachment to these movements, and you
do not open these parts and make them accept the Mother's
Light and Force to purify them. If you did that and,
instead of lamenting and getting troubled and clinging to
the idea that you cannot get rid of these things, insisted
quietly with a calm faith and patient resolution on their
disappearance, separating yourself from them, refusing to
accept them or at all regard them as part of yourself, they
would after a time lose their force and dwindle.

*

The sex-trouble is serious only so long as it can get the
consent of the mind and the vital will. If it is driven from
the mind, that is, if the mind refuses its consent, but the
vital part responds to it, it comes as a large wave of vital
desire and tries to sweep the mind away by force along
with it. If it is driven also from the higher vital, from the
heart and the dynamic possessive life-force, it takes refuge
in the lower vital and comes in the shape of smaller
suggestions and urges there. Driven from the lower vital

level, it goes down into the obscure inertly repetitive physical and comes as sensations in the sex-centre and a mechanical response to suggestion. Driven from there too, it goes down into the subconscient and comes up as dreams and night-emissions even without dreams. But to wherever it recedes, it tries still for a time from that base or refuge to trouble and recapture the assent of the higher parts, until the victory is complete and it is driven even out of the surrounding or environmental consciousness which is the extension of ourselves into the general or universal Nature.

*

When the psychic puts its influence on the vital, the first thing you must be careful to avoid is any least mixture of a wrong vital movement with the psychic movement. Lust is the perversion or degradation which prevents love from establishing its reign; so when there is the movement of psychic love in the heart, lust or vital desire is the one thing that must not be allowed to come in – just as when strength comes down from above, personal ambition and pride have to be kept far away from it; for any mixture of the perversion will corrupt the psychic or spiritual action and prevent a true fulfilment.

*

Pranayama and other physical practices like Asana do not necessarily root out sexual desire – sometimes by increasing enormously the vital force in the body they can even exaggerate in a rather startling way the force too of the sexual tendency, which, being at the base of the phy-

sical life, is always difficult to conquer. The one thing to
do is to separate oneself from these movements, to find
one's inner-self and live in it; these movements will not
then any longer appear as belonging to oneself but as
surface impositions of the outer Prakriti upon the inner
self or Purusha. They can then be more easily discarded or
brought to nothing.

*

This kind of sexual attack through sleep does not depend very much on food or anything else that is outward.
It is a mechanical habit in the subconscient; when the
sexual impulse is rejected or barred out in the waking
thoughts and feelings, it comes in this form in sleep, for
then there is only the subconscient at work and there is no
conscious control. It is a sign of sexual desire suppressed
in the waking mind and vital, but not eliminated in the
stuff of the physical nature.

To eliminate it one must first be careful to harbour no
sexual imagination or feeling in the waking state, next, to
put a strong will on the body and especially on the sexual
centre that there should be nothing of the kind in sleep.
This may not succeed at once, but if persevered in for a
long time, it usually has a result; the subconscient begins
to obey.

*

Hurting the flesh is no remedy for the sex-impulse,
though it may be a temporary diversion. It is the vital and
mostly the vital-physical that takes the sense-perception as
pleasure or otherwise.

Reduction of diet has not usually a permanent effect. It may give a greater sense of physical or vital-physical purity, lighten the system and reduce certain kinds of *tamas*. But the sex-impulse can very well accommodate itself to a reduced diet. It is not by physical means but by a change in the consciousness that these things can be surmounted.

*

Your difficulty in getting rid of the aboriginal in your nature will remain so long as you try to change your vital part by the sole or main strength of your mind and mental will, calling in at most an indefinite and impersonal divine power to aid you. It is an old difficulty which has never been radically solved in life itself because it has never been met in the true way. In many ways of yoga it does not so supremely matter because the aim is not a transformed life but withdrawal from life. When that is the object of an endeavour, it may be sufficient to keep the vital down by a mental and moral compulsion, or else it may be stilled and kept lying in a kind of sleep and quiescence. There are some even who allow it to run and exhaust itself if it can while its possessor professes to be untouched and unconcerned by it; for it is only old Nature running on by a past impetus and will drop off with the fall of the body. When none of these solutions can be attained, the sadhak sometimes simply leads a double inner life, divided between his spiritual experiences and his vital weaknesses to the end, making the most of his better part, making as little as may be of the outer being. But none of these methods will do for our purpose. If you want a true mastery and transformation of the vital movements, it can be done only on condition you allow your psychic being, the soul in you, to awake fully, to establish its rule and opening all to the permanent touch of the Divine Shakti, impose its own way of pure devotion, whole-hearted aspiration and complete uncompromising urge to all that is divine on the mind and heart and vital nature. There is no other way and it is no use hankering after a more comfortable path. *Nānyaḥ panthā vidyate ayanāya.*

V

PHYSICAL CONSCIOUSNESS – SUBCONSCIENT – SLEEP AND DREAM – ILLNESS

Our object is the supramental realisation and we have to do whatever is necessary for that or towards that under the conditions of each stage. At present the necessity is to prepare the physical consciousness; for that a complete equality and peace and a complete dedication free from personal demand or desire in the physical and the lower vital parts are the things to be established. Other things can come in their proper time. What is needed now is the psychic opening in the physical consciousness and the constant presence and guidance there.

*

What you describe is the material consciousness; it is mostly subconscient, but the part of it that is conscious is mechanical, inertly moved by habits or by the forces of the lower nature. Always repeating the same unintelligent and unenlightened movements, it is attached to the routine and established rule of what already exists, unwilling to change, unwilling to recieve the Light or obey the higher Force. Or, if it is willing, then it is unable. Or, if it is able, then it turns the action given to it by the Light or the Force into a new mechanical routine and so takes out of it all soul and life. It is obscure, stupid, indolent, full of ignorance and inertia, darkness and slowness of *tamas*.

It is this material consciousness into which we are seeking to bring first the higher (divine or spiritual) Light and

Power and Ananda, and then the Supramental Truth which is the object of our Yoga.

*

It is the most physical consciousness of which you have become aware; it is like that in almost everyone: when one gets fully or exclusively into it, one feels it to be like that of an animal, either obscure and restless or inert and stupid and in either condition not open to the Divine. It is only by bringing the Force and higher consciousness into it that it can fundamentally alter. When these things show themselves do not be upset by their emergence, but understand that they are there to be changed.

Here as elsewhere, quiet is the first thing needed, to keep the consciousness quiet, not allow it to get agitated and in turmoil. Then in the quiet to call for the Force to clear up all this obscurity and change it.

*

"At the mercy of the external sounds and external bodily sensations", "no control to drop the ordinary consciousness at will", "the whole tendency of the being away from Yoga" – all that is unmistakably applicable to the physical mind and the physical consciousness when they isolate themselves, as it were, and take up the whole front, pushing the rest into the background. When a part of the being is brought forward to be worked upon for change, this kind of all-occupying emergence, the dominant activity of that part as if it alone existed, very usually happens, and unfortunately it is always what has to be changed, the undesirable conditions, the difficulties of that part which rise first and obstinately hold the field and recur. In the physical it is inertia, obscurity, inability that come up and the obstinacy of these things. The only thing to do in this unpleasant phase is to be more obstinate than the physical inertia and to persist in a fixed endeavour – steady persistency without any restless struggle – to get a wide and permanent opening made even in this solid rock of obstruction.

*

These variations in the consciousness during the day are a thing that is common to almost everybody in the sadhana. The principle of oscillation, relaxation, relapse to a normal or a past lower condition from a higher state that is experienced but not yet perfectly stable, becomes very strong and marked when the working of the sadhana is in the physical consciousness. For there is an inertia in the physical nature that does not easily allow the intensity natural to the higher consciousness to remain constant, – the physical is always sinking back to something more ordinary; the higher consciousness and its force have to work long and come again and again before they can become constant and normal in the physical nature. Do not be disturbed or discouraged by these variations or this delay, however long and tedious; remain careful only to be quiet always with an inner quietude and as open as possible to the higher Power, not allowing any really adverse condition to get hold of you. If there is no adverse wave, then the rest is only a persistence of imperfections which all have in abundance; that imperfection and persistence the Force must work out and eliminate, but for the elimination time is needed.

*

You should not allow yourself to be discouraged by any persistence of the movements of the lower vital nature. There are some that tend always to persist and return until the whole physical nature is changed by the transformation of the most material consciousness; till then their pressure recurs – sometimes with a revival of their force, sometimes more dully – as a mechanical habit. Take from them all life-force by refusing any mental or vital assent; then the mechanical habit will become powerless to influence the thoughts and acts and will finally cease.

*

The Muladhar is the centre of the physical consciousness proper, and all below in the body is the sheer physical, which as it goes downward becomes increasingly subconscient, but the real seat of the subconscient is below the body, as the real seat of the higher consciousness (superconscient) is above the body. At the same time, the subconscient can be felt anywhere, felt as something below the movement of the consciousness and, in a way, supporting it from beneath or else drawing the consciousness down towards itself. The subconscient is the main support of all habitual movements, especially the physical and lower vital movements. When something is thrown out of the vital or physical, it very usually goes down into the subconscient and remains there as if in seed and comes up again when it can. That is the reason why it is so difficult to get rid of habitual vital movements or to change the character; for, supported or refreshed from this source, preserved in this matrix, your vital movements, even when suppressed or repressed, surge up again and recur. The action of the subconscient is irrational, mechanical, repetitive. It does not listen to reason or the mental will. It is only by bringing the higher Light and Force into it that it can change.

*

The subconscient is universal as well as individual like all the other main parts of the nature. But there are different parts or planes of the subconscient. All upon earth is based on the Inconscient as it is called, though it is not really inconscient at all, but rather a complete "sub"-conscience, a suppressed or involved consciousness, in which there is everything but nothing is formulated or expressed. The subconscient lies between this Inconscient and the conscious mind, life and body. It contains the potentiality of all the primitive reactions to life which struggle out to the surface from the dull and inert strands of Matter and form by a constant development a slowly evolving and self-formulating consciousness; it contains them not as ideas, perceptions or conscious reactions but as fluid substance of these things. But also all that is consciously experienced sinks down into the subconscient, not as precise though submerged memories but as obscure yet obstinate impressions of experience, and these can come up at any time as dreams, as mechanical repetitions of past thought, feelings, action, etc., as "complexes" exploding into action and event, etc., etc. The subconscient is the main cause why all things repeat themselves and nothing ever gets changed except in appearance. It is the cause why people say character cannot be changed, the cause also of the constant return of things one hoped to have got rid of for ever. All seeds are there and all Samskaras of the mind, vital and body, – it is the main support of death and disease and the last fortress (seemingly impregnable) of the Ignorance. All too that is suppressed without being wholly got rid of sinks down there and remains as seed ready to surge up or sprout up at any moment.

*

The subconscious is the evolutionary basis in us, it is not the whole of our hidden nature, nor is it the whole origin of what we are. But things can rise from the subconscient and take shape in the conscious parts and much of our smaller vital and physical instincts, movements, habits, character-forms has this source.

There are three occult sources of our action – the superconscient, the subliminal, the subconscient, but of none of them are we in control or even aware. What we are aware of is the surface being which is only an instrumental arrangement. The source of all is the general Nature, – universal Nature individualising itself in each person; for this general Nature deposits certain habits of movement, personality, character, faculties, dispositions, tendencies in us, and that, whether formed now or before our birth, is what we usually call ourselves. A good deal of this is in habitual movement and use in our known conscious parts on the surface, a great deal more is concealed in the other unknown three which are below or behind the surface.

But what we are on the surface is being constantly set in motion, changed, developed or repeated by the waves of the general Nature coming in on us either directly or else indirectly through others, through circumstances, through various agencies or channels. Some of this flows straight into the conscious parts and acts there, but our mind ignores its source, appropriates it and regards all that as its own; a part comes secretly into the subconscient or sinks into it and waits for an opportunity of rising up into the conscious surface; a good deal goes into the subliminal and may at any time come out – or may not, may rather rest there as unused matter. Part passes through and is rejected, thrown back or thrown out or spilt into the universal sea. Our nature is a constant activity of forces supplied to us out of which (or rather out of a small amount of it) we make what we will or can. What we make seems fixed and formed for good, but in reality it is all a play of forces, a flux, nothing fixed or stable; the appearance of stability is given by constant repetition and recurrence of the same vibrations and formations. That is why our nature can be changed in spite of Vivekananda's saying and Horace's adage and in spite of the conservative resistance of the subconscient, but it is a difficult job because the master mode of Nature is this obstinate repetition and recurrence.

As for the things in our nature that are thrown away from us by rejection but come back, it depends on where you throw them. Very often there is a sort of procedure about it. The mind rejects its mentalities, the vital its vitalities, the physical its physicalities – these usually go back into the corresponding domain of general Nature. It all stays at first, when that happens, in the environmental consciousness which we carry about with us, by which we communicate with the outside Nature, and often it persistently rushes back from there – until it is so absolutely rejected, or thrown far away as it were, that it cannot return upon us any more. But when what the thinking and willing mind rejects is strongly supported by the vital, it leaves the mind indeed but sinks down into the vital, rages

there and tries to rush up again and re-occupy the mind
and compel or capture our mental acceptance. When the
higher vital too – the heart or the larger vital dynamis
reject it, it sinks from there and takes refuge in the lower
vital with its mass of small current movements that make
up our daily littleness. When the lower vital too rejects it,
it sinks into the physical consciousness and tries to stick by
inertia or mechanical repetition. Rejected even from
there it goes into the subconscient and comes up in dreams,
in passivity, in extreme *tamas*. The Inconscient is the last
resort of the Ignorance.

As for the waves that recur from the general Nature, it
is the natural tendency of the inferior forces there to try
and perpetuate their action in the individual, to rebuild
what he has unbuilt of their deposits in him; so they return
on him, often with an increased force, even with a stu-
pendous violence, when they find their influence rejected.
But they cannot last long once the environmental consciousness is cleared – unless the "Hostiles" take a hand.
Even then these can indeed attack, but if the sadhak has
established his position in the inner self, they can only
attack and retire.

It is true that we bring most of ourselves, – or rather
most of our predispositions, tendencies of reaction to the
universal Nature, from past lives. Heredity only affects
strongly the external being; besides, all the effects of
heredity are not accepted even there, only those that are
in consonance with what we are to be or not preventive of
it at least.

*

The subconscient is a thing of habits and memories and

repeats persistently or whenever it can old suppressed reactions, reflexes, mental, vital or physical responses. It must be trained by a still more persistent insistence of the higher parts of the being to give up its old responses and take on the new and true ones.

*

You do not realise how much of the ordinary natural being lives in the subconscient physical. It is there that habitual movements, mental and vital, are stored and from there they come up into the waking mind. Driven out of the upper consciousness, it is in this cavern of the Panis that they take refuge. No longer allowed to emerge freely in the waking state, they come up in sleep as dreams. It is when they are cleared out of the subconscient, their very seeds killed by the enlightening of these hidden layers, that they cease for good. As your consciousness deepens inwardly and the higher light comes down into those inferior covered parts, the things that now recur in this way will disappear.

*

It is certainly possible to draw forces from below. It may be the hidden divine forces from below that rise at your pull, and then this motion upward completes the motion and effort of the divine force from above, helping especially to bring it into the body. Or it may be the obscure forces from below that respond to the summons and then this kind of drawing brings either *tamas* or disturbance – sometimes great masses of inertia or a formidable up-heaval and disturbance.

The lower vital is a very obscure plane and it can be fully opened with advantage only when the other planes above it have been thrown wide to light and knowledge. One who concentrates on the lower vital without that higher preparation and without knowledge is likely to fall into many confusions. This does not mean that experiences of this plane may not come earlier or even at the beginning; they do come of themselves, but they must not be given too large a place.

*

There is a Yoga-Shakti lying coiled or asleep in the inner body, not active. When one does Yoga, this force uncoils itself and rises upward to meet the Divine Consciousness and force that are waiting above us. When this happens, when the awakened Yoga-Shakti arises, it is often felt like a snake uncoiling and standing up straight and lifting itself more and more upwards. When it meets the Divine Consciousness above, then the force of the Divine Consciousness can more easily descend into the body and be felt working there to change the nature.

The feeling of your body and eyes being drawn upwards is part of the same movement. It is the inner consciousness in the body and the inner subtle sight in the body that are looking and moving upward and trying to meet the divine consciousness and divine seeing above.

*

If you go down into your lower parts or ranges of nature, you must be always careful to keep a vigilant connection with the higher already regenerated levels of the consciousness and to bring down the Light and Purity through them into these nether still unregenerated regions. If there is not this vigilance, one gets absorbed in the unregenerated movement of the inferior layers and there is obscuration and trouble.

The safest way is to remain in the higher part of the consciousness and put a pressure from it on the lower to change. It can be done in this way, only you must get the knack and the habit of it. If you achieve the power to do that, it makes the progress much easier, smoother and less painful.

*

Your practice of psycho-analysis was a mistake. It has for the time at least, made the work of purification more complicated, not easier. The psycho-analysis of Freud is the last thing that one should associate with Yoga. It takes up a certain part, the darkest, the most perilous, the unhealthiest part of the nature, the lower vital subconscious layer, isolates some of its most morbid phenomena and attributes to it and them an action out of all proportion to its true role in the nature. Modern psychology is an infant science, at once rash, fumbling and crude. As in all infant sciences, the universal habit of the human mind – to take a partial or local truth, generalise it unduly and try to explain a whole field of nature in its narrow terms – runs riot here. Moreover, the exaggeration of the importance of suppressed sexual complexes is a dangerous falsehood and it can have a nasty influence and tend to make the mind and vital more and not less fundamentally impure than before.

It is true that the subliminal in man is the largest part of his nature and has in it the secret of the unseen dynamisms which explain his surface activities. But the lower vital subconscious which is all that this psycho-analysis of Freud seems to know – and even of that it knows only a few ill-lit corners, – is no more than a restricted and very inferior portion of the subliminal whole. The subliminal self stands behind and supports the whole superficial man; it has in it a larger and more efficient mind behind the surface mind, a larger and more powerful vital behind the surface vital, a subtler and freer physical consciousness behind the surface bodily existence. And above them it opens to higher superconscient as well as below them to lower subconscient ranges. If one wishes to purify and transform the nature, it is the power of these higher ranges to which one must open and raise to them and change by them both the subliminal and the surface being. Even this should be done with care, not prematurely or rashly, following a higher guidance, keeping always the right attitude; for otherwise the force that is drawn down may be too strong for an obscure and weak frame of nature. But to begin by opening up the lower subconscious, risking to raise up all that is foul or obscure in it, is to go out of one's way to invite trouble. First, one should make the higher mind and vital strong and firm and full of light and peace from above; afterwards one can open up or even dive into the subconscious with more safety and some chance of a rapid and successful change.

The system of getting rid of things by *anubhava* can also be a dangerous one; for on this way one can easily become more entangled instead of arriving at freedom. This method has behind it two well-known psychological motives. One, the motive of purposeful exhaustion, is valid only in some cases, especially when some natural tendency has too strong a hold or too strong a drive in it to be got rid of by *vicāra* or by the process of rejection and the substitution of the true movement in its place; when that happens in excess, the sadhak has sometimes even to go back to the ordinary action of the ordinary life, get the true experience of it with a new mind and will behind and then return to the spiritual life with the obstacle eliminated or else ready for elimination. But this method of purposive indulgence is always dangerous, though sometimes inevitable. It succeeds only when there is a very strong will in the being towards realisation; for then indulgence brings a strong dissatisfaction and reaction, *vairagya*, and the will towards perfection can be carried down into the recalcitrant part of the nature.

The other motive for *anubhava* is of a more general applicability; for in order to reject anything from the being one has first to become conscious of it, to have the clear inner experience of its action and to discover its actual place in the workings of the nature. One can then work upon it to eliminate it, if it is an entirely wrong movement, or to transform it if it is only the degradation of a higher and true movement. It is this or something like it that is attempted crudely and improperly with a rudimentary and insufficient knowledge in the system of psycho-analysis. The process of raising up the lower movements into the full light of consciousness in order to know and deal with them is inevitable; for there can be no complete change without it. But it can truly succeed only when a higher light and force are sufficiently at work to overcome, sooner or later, the force of the tendency that is held up for change. Many, under the pretext of *anubhava*, not only raise up the adverse movement, but support it with their consent instead of rejecting it, find

justifications for continuing or repeating it and so go on
playing with it, indulging its return, eternising it; afterwards when they want to get rid of it, it has got such a hold
that they find themselves helpless in its clutch and only a
terrible struggle or an intervention of divine grace can
liberate them. Some do this out of a vital twist or perver-
sity, others out of sheer ignorance; but in Yoga, as in life,
ignorance is not accepted by Nature as a justifying excuse.
This danger is there in all improper dealings with the
ignorant parts of the nature; but none is more ignorant,
more perilous, more unreasoning and obstinate in recurrence than the lower vital subconscious and its movements.
To raise it up prematurely or improperly for *anubhava* is
to risk suffusing the conscious parts also with its dark and
dirty stuff and thus poisoning the whole vital and even the
mental nature. Always therefore one should begin by a
positive, not a negative experience, by bringing down
something of the divine nature, calm, light, equanimity,
purity, divine strength into the parts of the conscious
being that have to be changed; only when that has been
sufficiently done and there is a firm positive basis, is it safe
to raise up the concealed subconscious adverse elements
in order to destroy and eliminate them by the strength of
the divine calm, light, force and knowledge. Even so,
there will be enough of the lower stuff rising up of itself to
give you as much of the *anubhava* as you will need for
getting rid of the obstacles; but then they can be dealt with
with much less danger and under a higher internal guidance.

*

I find it difficult to take these psycho-analysts at all

seriously when they try to scrutinise spiritual experience
by the flicker of their torch-lights, – yet perhaps one ought
to, for half-knowledge is a powerful thing and can be a
great obstacle to the coming in front of the true Truth.
This new psychology looks to me very much like children
learning some summary and not very adequate alphabet,
exulting in putting their a-b-c-d of the subconscient and
the mysterious underground super-ego together and
imagining that their first book of obscure beginnings (c-a-t
cat, t-r-e-e tree) is the very heart of the real knowledge.
They look from down up and explain the higher lights by
the lower obscurities; but the foundation of these things is
above and not below, *upari budhna eṣām*. The superconscient, not the subconscient, is the true foundation of
things. The significance of the lotus is not to be found by
analysing the secrets of the mud from which it grows here;
its secret is to be found in the heavenly archetype of the
lotus that blooms for ever in the Light above. The self-
chosen field of these psychologists is besides poor, dark
and limited; you must know the whole before you can
know the part and the highest before you can truly understand the lowest. That is the promise of the greater psychology awaiting its hour before which these poor gropings
will disappear and come to nothing.

*

Sleep, because of its subconscient basis, usually brings a
falling down to a lower level, unless it is a conscious sleep;
to make it more and more conscious is the one permanent
remedy: but also until that is done, one should always
react against this sinking tendency when one wakes and
not allow the effect of dull nights to accumulate. But these

things need always a settled endeavour and discipline and must take time, sometimes a long time. It will not do to refrain from the effort because immediate results do not appear.

*

The consciousness in the night almost always descends below the level of what one has gained by sadhana in the waking consciousness, unless there are special experiences of an uplifting character in the time of sleep or unless the Yogic consciousness acquired is so strong in the physical itself as to counteract the pull of the subconscient inertia. In ordinary sleep the consciousness in the body is that of the subconscient physical, which is a diminished consciousness, not awake and alive like the rest of the being. The rest of the being stands back and part of its consciousness goes out into other planes and regions and has experiences which are recorded in dreams such as that you have related. You say you go to very bad places and have experiences like the one you narrate; but that is not a sign, necessarily, of anything wrong in you. It merely means that you go into the vital world, as everybody does, and the vital world is full of such places and such experiences. What you have to do is not so much to avoid at all going there, for it cannot be avoided altogether, but to go with full protection until you get mastery in these regions of supra-physical Nature. That is one reason why you should remember the Mother and open to the Force before sleeping; for the more you get that habit and do it successfully, the more the protection will be with you.

*

These dreams are not all mere dreams, all have not a casual, incoherent or subconscious building. Many are records or transcripts of experiences on the vital plane into which one enters in sleep, some are scenes or events of the subtle physical plane. There one often undergoes happenings or carries on actions that resemble those of the physical life with the same surroundings and the same people, though usually there is in arrangement and feature some or a considerable difference. But it may also be a contact with other surroundings and with other people, not known in the physical life or not belonging at all to the physical world.

In the waking state you are conscious only of a certain limited field and action of your nature. In sleep you can become vividly aware of things beyond this field – a larger mental or vital nature behind the waking state or else a subtle physical or a subconscient nature which contains much that is there in you but not distinguishably active in the waking state. All these obscure tracts have to be cleared or else there can be no change of Prakriti. You should not allow yourself to be disturbed by the press of vital or subconscient dreams – for these two make up the larger part of dream-experience – but aspire to get rid of these things and of the activities they indicate, to be conscious and reject all but the divine Truth; the more you get that Truth and cling to it in the waking state, rejecting all else, the more all this inferior dream-stuff will get clear.

*

The dreams you describe are very clearly symbolic dreams on the vital plane. These dreams may symbolise anything, forces at play, the underlying structure and tissue of things done or experienced, actual or potential happenings, real or suggested movements or changes in the inner or outer nature.

The timidity of which the apprehension in the dream was an indication, was probably not anything in the conscious mind or higher vital, but something subconscient in the lower vital nature. This part always feels itself small and insignificant and has very easily a fear of being submerged by the greater consciousness – a fear which in some may amount at the first contact to something like a panic, alarm or terror.

*

All dreams of this kind are very obviously formations such as one often meets on the vital, more rarely on the mental plane. Sometimes they are the formations of your own mind or vital; sometimes they are the formations of other minds with an exact or modified transcription in yours; sometimes formations come that are made by the non-human forces or beings of these other planes. These things are not true and need not become true in the physical world, but they may still have effects on the physical if they are framed with that purpose or that tendency and, if they are allowed, they may realise their events or their meaning – for they are most often symbolical or schematic – in the inner or the outer life. The proper course with them is simply to observe and understand and, if they are from a hostile source, reject or destroy them.

There are other dreams that have not the same character but are a representation or transcription of things that actually happen on other planes, in other worlds, under other conditions than ours. There are, again, some dreams that are purely symbolic and some that indicate existing movements and propensities in us, whether familiar or undetected by the waking mind, or exploit old memories or else raise up things either passively stored or still active in the subconscient, a mass of various stuff which has to be changed or got rid of as one rises into a higher consciousness. If one learns how to interpret, one can get from dreams much knowledge of the secrets of our nature and of other-nature.

*

It is not a right method to try to keep awake at night; the suppression of the needed sleep makes the body *tāmasic* and unfit for the necessary concentration during the waking hours. The right way is to transform the sleep and not suppress it, and especially to learn how to become more and more conscious in sleep itself. If that is done, sleep changes into an inner mode of consciousness in which the sadhana can continue as much as in the waking state, and at the same time one is able to enter into other planes of consciousness than the physical and command an immense range of informative and utilisable experience.

*

Sleep cannot be replaced, but it can be changed; for you can become conscious in sleep. If you are thus conscious, then the night can be utilised for a higher working – provided the body gets its due rest; for the object of sleep is the body's rest and the renewal of the vital-physical force. It is a mistake to deny to the body food and sleep, as some from an ascetic idea or impulse want to do – that only wears out the physical support and although either the Yogic or the vital energy can long keep at work an over-strained or declining physical system, a time comes when this drawing is no longer so easy nor perhaps possible. The body should be given what it needs for its own efficient working. Moderate but sufficient food (without greed or desire), sufficient sleep, but not of the heavy *tāmasic* kind, this should be the rule.

*

The sleep you describe in which there is a luminous silence or else the sleep in which there is Ananda in the cells, these are obviously the best states. The other hours, those of which you are unconscious, may be spells of a deep slumber in which you have got out of the physical into the mental, vital or other planes. You say you were unconscious, but it may simply be that you do not remember what happened; for in coming back there is a sort of turning over of the consciousness, a transition or reversal, in which everything experienced in sleep except perhaps the last happening of all or else one that was very impressive, recedes from the physical consciousness and all becomes as if a blank. There is another blank state, a state of inertia, not only blank, but heavy and unremembering; but that is when one goes deeply and crassly into the subconscient; this subterranean plunge is very undesirable, obscuring, lowering, often fatiguing rather than restful, the reverse of the luminous silence.

*

It was not half sleep or quarter sleep or even one-sixteenth sleep that you had; it was a going inside of the consciousness, which in that state remains conscious but shut to outer things and open only to inner experience. You must distinguish clearly between these two quite different conditions, one is *nidra*, the other, the beginning at least of *samadhi* (not *nirvikalpa*, of course). This drawing inside is necessary because the active mind of the human being is at first too much turned to outward things; it has to go inside altogether in order to live in the inner being (inner mind, inner vital, inner physical, psychic). But with training one can arrive at a point when one remains outwardly conscious and yet lives in the inner being and has at will the indrawn or the outpoured condition; you can then have the same dense immobility and the same inpouring of a greater and purer consciousness in the waking state as in that which you erroneously call sleep.

*

Physical fatigue like this in the course of the sadhana may come from various reasons:

(*i*) It may come from receiving more than the physical is ready to assimilate. The cure is then quiet rest in conscious immobility receiving the forces but not for any other purpose than the recuperation of the strength and energy.

(*ii*) It may be due to the passivity taking the form of inertia – inertia brings the consciousness down towards the ordinary physical level which is soon fatigued and prone to *tamas*. The cure here is to get back into the true consciousness and to rest there, not in inertia.

(*iii*) It may be due to mere overstrain of the body – not

giving it enough sleep or repose. The body is the support
of the Yoga, but its energy is not inexhaustible and needs
to be husbanded, it can be kept up by drawing on the
universal vital Force but that reinforcement too has its
limits. A certain moderation is needed even in the eagerness for progress – moderation, not indifference or indolence.

*

Illness marks some imperfection or weakness or else
opening to adverse touches in the physical nature and is
often connected also with some obscurity or disharmony
in the lower vital or the physical mind or elsewhere.

It is very good if one can get rid of illness entirely by
faith and Yoga-power or the influx of the Divine Force.
But very often this is not altogether possible, because the
whole nature is not open or able to respond to the Force.
The mind may have faith and respond, but the lower vital
and the body may not follow. Or, if the mind and vital are
ready, the body may not respond, or may respond only
partially, because it has the habit of replying to the forces
which produce a particular illness, and habit is a very
obstinate force in the material part of the nature. In such
cases the use of the physical means can be resorted to, –
not as the main means, but as a help or material support to
the action of the Force. Not strong and violent remedies,
but those that are beneficial without disturbing the body.

*

Attacks of illness are attacks of the lower nature or of
adverse forces taking advantage of some weakness, opening or response in the nature, – like all other things that

come and have got to be thrown away, they come from
outside. If one can feel them so coming and get the
strength and the habit to throw them away before they can
enter the body, then one can remain free from illness.
Even when the attack seems to rise from within, that
means only that it has not been detected before it entered
the subconscient; once in the subconscient, the force that
brought it rouses it from there sooner or later and it
invades the system. When you feel it just after it has
entered, it is because though it came direct and not
through the subconscient, yet you could not detect it while
it was still outside. Very often it arrives like that frontally
or more often tangentially from the side direct, forcing its
way through the subtle vital envelope which is our main
armour of defense, but it can be stopped there in the
envelope itself before it penetrates the material body.
Then one may feel some effect, *e.g.,* feverishness or a
tendency to cold, but there is not the full invasion of the
malady. If it can be stopped earlier or if the vital envelope
of itself resists and remains strong, vigorous and intact,
then there is no illness; the attack produces no physical
effect and leaves no traces.

*

Certainly, one can act from within on an illness and cure
it. Only it is not always easy as there is much resistance in
Matter, a resistance of inertia. An untiring persistence is
necessary; at first one may fail altogether or the symptoms
increase, but gradually the control of the body or of a
particular illness becomes stronger. Again, to cure an
occasional attack of illness by inner means is comparatively easy, to make the body immune from it in future is

more difficult. A chronic malady is harder to deal with, more reluctant to disappear entirely than an occasional disturbance of the body. So long as the control of the body is imperfect, there are all these and other imperfections and difficulties in the use of the inner force.

If you can succeed by the inner action in preventing increase, even that is something; you have then by *abhyāsa* to strengthen the power till it becomes able to cure. Note that so long as the power is not entirely there, some aid of physical means need not be altogether rejected.

*

Medicines are a *pis aller* that have to be used when something in the consciousness does not respond or responds superficially to the Force. Very often it is some part of the material consciousness that is unreceptive – at other times it is the subconscient which stands in the way even when the whole waking mind, life, physical consent to the liberating influence. If the subconscient also answers, then even a slight touch of the Force can not only cure the particular illness but make that form or kind of illness practically impossible hereafter.

*

Your theory of illness is rather a perilous creed – for illness is a thing to be eliminated, not accepted or enjoyed. There *is* something in the being that enjoys illness, it is possible even to turn the pains of illness like any other pain into a form of pleasure; for pain and pleasure are both of them degradations of an original Ananda and can be reduced into terms of each other or else sublimated into their original principle of Ananda. It is true also that one must be able to bear illness with calm, equanimity, endurance, even recognition of it, since it has come, as something that had to be passed through in the course of experience. But to accept and enjoy it means to help it to last and that will not do; for illness is a deformation of the physical nature just as lust, anger, jealousy, etc., are deformations of the vital nature and error and prejudice and indulgence of falsehood are deformations of the mental nature. All these things have to be eliminated and rejection is the first condition of their disappearance while acceptance has a contrary effect altogether.

*

All illnesses pass through the nervous or vital-physical sheath of the subtle consciousness and subtle body before they enter the physical. If one is conscious of the subtle body or with the subtle consciousness, one can stop an illness on its way and prevent it from entering the physical body. But it may have come without one's noticing, or when one is asleep or through the subconscient, or in a sudden rush when one is off one's guard; then there is nothing to do but to fight it out from a hold already gained on the body. Self-defence by these inner means may become so strong that the body becomes practically immune as many Yogis are. Still this "practically" does not mean "absolutely". The absolute immunity can only come with the supramental change. For below the supramental it is the result of an action of a Force among many forces and can be disturbed by a disruption of the equilibrium established – in the supramental it is a law of the nature; in a supramentalised body immunity from illness would be automatic, inherent in its new nature.

There is a difference between Yogic Force on the mental and inferior planes and the Supramental Nature. What is acquired and held by the Yoga-Force in the mind-and-body consciousness is in the supramental inherent and exists not by achievement but by nature – it is self-existent and absolute.